POSITIONING IN A WHEELCHAIR

A Guide for Professional Caregivers of the Disabled Adult

Jan K. Mayall, Dip PT/OT
Guylaine Desharnais, BSc, OTR

SLACK Incorporated, 6900 Grove Road, Thorofare, New Jersey 08086

SLACK International Book Distributors

Japan
  Igaku-Shoin, Ltd.
  Tokyo International P.O. Box 5063
  1-28-36 Hongo, Bunkyo-Ku
  Tokyo 113
  Japan

Australia
  McGraw-Hill Book Company
  4 Barcoo Street
  Roseville East 2069
  New South Wales
  Australia

Canada
  McGraw-Hill Ryerson Limited
  300 Water Street
  Whitby, Ontario
  L1N 9B6
  Canada

United Kingdom
  McGraw-Hill Book Company
  Shoppenhangers Road
  Maidenhead, Berkshire SL6 2QL
  England

In all other regions throughout the world, SLACK professional reference books are available through offices and affiliates of McGraw-Hill, Inc. For the name and address of the office serving your area, please correspond to

  McGraw-Hill, Inc.
  Medical Publishing Group
  Attn: International Marketing Director
  1221 Avenue of the Americas —28th Floor
  New York, NY 10020
  (212)-512-3955 (phone)
  (212)-512-4717 (fax)

Editorial Director: Cheryl D. Willoughby
Publisher: Harry C. Benson

Printed in the United States of America

Library of Congress Catalog Card Number: 89-43139

ISBN: 1-55642-147-8

Published by: SLACK Incorporated
               6900 Grove Road
               Thorofare, NJ 08086-9447

Last digit is print number: 10 9 8 7 6 5 4 3 2

Contents

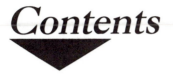

Acknowledgement

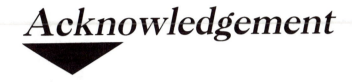

The authors wish to acknowledge with sincere gratitude Hughes Bernier for the drawings, Gaetan Laurendeau for the photography, Hazel Broadley for her assistance with editing this manuscript, and the residents of Banfield Pavilion, Vancouver General Hospital, for their patience as we learned and grew together.

Introduction

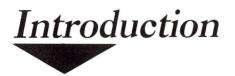

Many older disabled adults sit for hours each day, slumped over in wheelchairs which are designed primarily for transportation. Prolonged periods of sitting in such wheelchairs may not only be uncomfortable, but could pose multiple health hazards.

Positioning is a major concern to the occupational therapist working with clients in long-term care. In many facilities, staff resources, material, and funding are limited, and positioning of the client in the wheelchair is not a priority. With increased attention to the position of the client, many costly interventions may be avoided, and the maintenance of independence and quality of life will be optimal.

The purpose of this manual is to provide caregivers with the knowledge of various techniques and appliances currently available that will optimize seating comfort and positioning of the older disabled adult with mild to moderate positioning problems. Primarily intended for use in long-term care settings, the information will also be useful for caregivers in the community. Severely impaired clients may require the services of a specialized seating clinic for a customized seating insert.

In using this manual, it may be tempting to turn directly to the possible solutions in order to deal with a specific problem. The reader is advised to make a thorough assessment of the problem before seeking a solution. Using a systematic approach to positioning should then provide a clear understanding of how to proceed.

Objectives

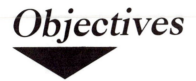

This manual is intended to assure optimal quality of life for the older disabled adult by meeting the following objectives:

—Maximizing participation and independence in performing activities of daily living
—Promoting the ability to interact with the environment
—Preventing pressure sores and alleviation of pain
—Preventing deformities
—Providing comfort
—Facilitating transfers and mobility
—Assuring safety.

Ideally, a client would be positioned to meet all of the above objectives. However, such a situation is seldom the case due to nonacceptance of a device by the client, limited financial resources, or other factors. The role of the caregiver is to ensure that all potential problems are addressed and the best possible solutions determined.

1
The Importance of Positioning

Sitting is a dynamic, not a static, behavior. When seated, many different postures are assumed, and vary according to the activity performed.

Good positioning in a wheelchair will contribute to general comfort, function, and well-being. The following are examples of how function is affected by positioning:

—When the head droops forward onto the chest, eating becomes difficult, and social and environmental interactions are minimal.

—Mobilizing the wheelchair is very difficult when one foot constantly falls off the footrest and drags on the floor.

—Use of the hands and arms is limited if the client has a weak trunk and leans to one side.

". . . good posture positively correlates not only with the integrity of joints, but also with the abilities to experience emotion appropriately, display sound, perceptual ability, and experience healthy organic functioning. Since posture has been demonstrated to be a variable in both mental and physical health, the maintenance of good posture should be a priority concern in institutions."[1]

Encouraging the older disabled adult to be up out of bed daily will lessen the hazard of immobility. The ability to shift position in the wheelchair is a safeguard against the possibility of pressure sores, contractures, loss of sensation, muscle atrophy, and other potential problems. These factors must be taken into consideration when positioning a client. The caregivers must be even more alert when there is lack of independent mobility. (Refer to Fig. 1-1)

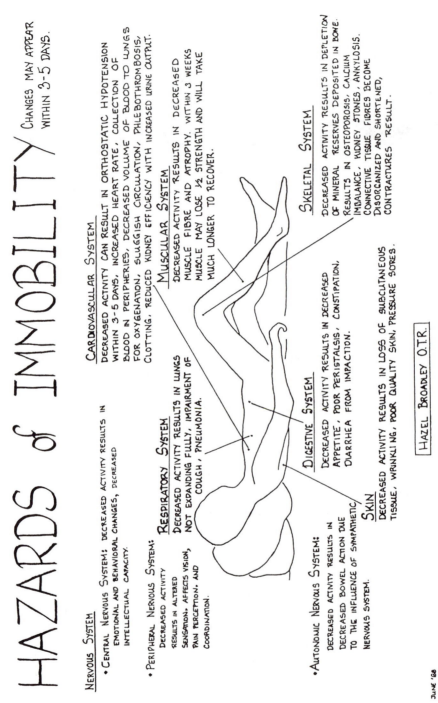

Figure 1-1.

2 ▼ Basic Position in a Wheelchair

There are two determining factors which affect the basic seating position, and they are of equal significance. The first is the selection of the correct size of wheelchair. The second is the use of a systematic approach to positioning. The systematic approach begins with the position of the pelvis; followed by the lower extremities from proximal to distal; the lower trunk; the upper trunk; the head and neck; and lastly, the upper extremities from proximal to distal.

Pelvis

The pelvis provides a stable base, the position of which forms the foundation for the support of the rest of the body.

The hips are positioned in the middle and as far back on the seat as possible so that the pelvis is centered and level. Check to see that the iliac crests are level and aligned from side to side to insure that there is no lateral rotation of the pelvis. The pelvis should be in a neutral position, i.e., not tilted forward or back excessively. The seat width must allow a 1.25 cm. (0.5 in.) clearance on each side. This helps distribute the weight over the widest possible surface and still allows for support of the trunk and upper extremities. Seat depth should allow a 5 cm.-7.5 cm.(2–3 in.) clearance from the back of the knee to the front of the sling seat. This is to distribute the weight evenly along the buttocks and thighs.

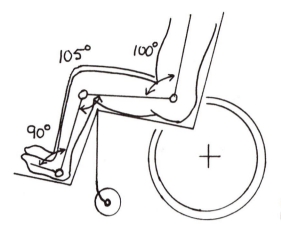

Figure 2-1. Position of lower extremities.

Lower Extremities

When adjusting the foot rest height, the client should be sitting on a cushion and wearing a pair of shoes or slippers. To check for good leg support, two fingers can be inserted under the thigh from the front of the cushion. They should slip in easily for 5 cm. (2 in.). The femurs should be parallel to the seat. This will encourage weight distribution from the coccyx-ischium region onto the well- padded thighs. The footrests should have at least a 5 cm. (2 in.) clearance from the floor. When the client is well positioned, the hips will be at about 100 degrees, the knees at 105 degrees and the ankles at 90 degrees with the heel resting flat on the footrests (Refer to Fig. 2-1).

Trunk

The height of the backrest depends on the amount of trunk support required. To check for adequate back support for clients with adequate trunk control,

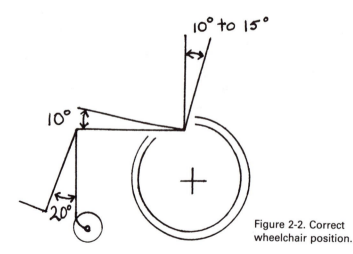

Figure 2-2. Correct wheelchair position.

insert the breadth of four fingers (about 10 cm. or 4 in.) between the top of the back upholstery to under the axilla.

Head and Neck

The head should be upright, supported by the neck in the mid-position.

Upper Extremities

For correct arm rest height, measure from the seat cushion to just under the elbow, which should be held at a right angle. Add 2.5 cm. (1 in.). Correct armrest height will help the client maintain good posture and balance. Comfortable support will also be provided to the upper extremities and shoulders.

Ideally, the wheelchair seat should be inclined toward the back by 10 degrees, the legs should be 20 degree from vertical, and the back 10 to 15 degrees from vertical. (Refer to Fig. 2-2)

3
Types of Wheelchairs

A wheelchair should assure comfort, independence, and an active life. It is necessary to be well informed about available products since there is a wide variety of wheelchairs on the market. A good understanding of the basic seating position will help determine the most appropriate type of wheelchair.

The following is a short description of a few types of wheelchairs which are in common use.

Standard Adult Wheelchair

—Regular adult: seat width 46 cm. (18 in.), seat height from floor 50 cm. (19.75 in.)
—Narrow adult: seat width 41 cm. (16 in.), seat height from floor 50 cm. (19.75 in.)

Hemi Wheelchair

—Available in Regular or Narrow Adult
—Seat height from floor is 44 cm. (17.50 in.), allowing the client to mobilize the wheelchair with one or both lower extremities.

Semi-reclining Wheelchair

—Wheelchair back reclines 30 degrees from vertical and locks in several positions

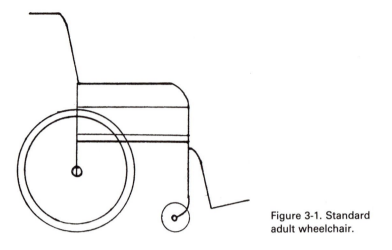

Figure 3-1. Standard
adult wheelchair.

—Back upholstery is higher than a standard adult wheelchair by 13 cm. (5 in.)
—Has a detachable 25 cm. (10 in.) telescopic headrest
—Rear wheels are set back 3 cm. (1.25 in.) to maintain good balance and stability of the wheelchair.

Fully-reclining Wheelchair

—Wheelchair back reclines to horizontal from vertical position and locks into various positions of recline
—Back upholstery is higher than a standard adult wheelchair by 17 cm. (7 in.)
—Has a detachable 25 cm. (10 in.) telescopic headrest

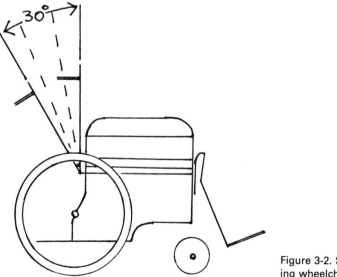

Figure 3-2. Semi-reclin-
ing wheelchair.

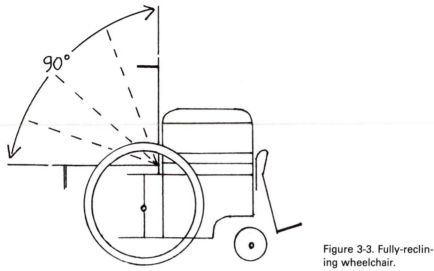

Figure 3-3. Fully-reclining wheelchair.

—Rear wheels are set back 12 cm. (5 in.) to maintain stability of the wheelchair.

Amputee Wheelchair

—Same width and height as standard adult wheelchair
—Rear wheel set back 3 cm. (1.25 in.) to maintain chair stability and to compensate for the loss of the lower extremity(ies)
—If an amputee wheelchair is not available:
  1. an amputee adapter (Everest and Jennings) can be adjusted to a standard adult wheelchair.

    or

  2. add 4.5 to 9 kilos (10 to 20 pounds) of weight to the foot rests.

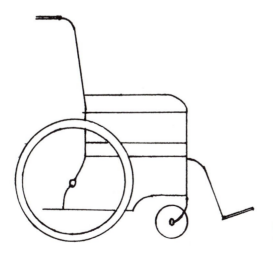

Figure 3-4. Amputee wheelchair.

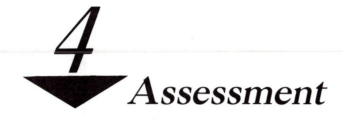

4 Assessment

Before deciding on the most appropriate positioning, a thorough assessment of the client is necessary. The information obtained from the assessment will determine:

—The problem
—The cause of the problem
—The objectives of positioning

The assessment should include:

- Diagnosis and prognosis
- Age
- Cognitive function:
  —memory
  —learning ability
  —comprehension
  —judgement
- Perceptual function, such as:
  —heminegligence
  —hemianopsia
  —apraxia
- Physical ability:
  —range of motion
  —muscle tone
  —strength
  —pain

- —contractures
- —sitting tolerance and balance
- Level of independence in activities of daily living.
- Transfer ability and modality.
- Mobility:
  - —ambulation
  - —wheelchair mobility
- Body weight
- Sensory status:
  - —vision
  - —hearing
  - —touch. A careful assessment of any area of impaired or absent sensation over the bony prominence, such as the ischial tuberosities, must be included.
- Presence of edema in lower and/or upper extremities.
- Skin integrity. How often is it checked? By whom? Is there a history of pressure sores, allergies, or a skin graft?
- Leisure interests and life style. Indoor/outdoor activities.
- Transportation to and from place of residence.
- Client usage of wheelchair. Is the client careless or rough on wheelchair?
- Amount of time spent daily in the wheelchair.
- Financial resources of the client.

The client must be involved in the whole process of wheelchair positioning, starting with the assessment. The caregiver needs to be sensitive to the priorities of the client and include them in the data collected.

For example: "Cosmesis, an important aspect of seating, is sometimes overlooked by therapists. For example, the choice of covering can be very important to families, even if it is not very important to the provision of seating. The seating system should be considered an extension of the client's tastes and self-image. If it meets only the needs of the provider, in terms of useability and appearance, the system will likely be used little."[10]

By allowing time for the understanding of the benefits of proper positioning, the client will often more readily accept the positioning technique or device used.

The primary caregivers, such as family members and nursing staff, have invaluable information to share since they spend the most time with the client. They should be consulted frequently during the assessment to assist in establishing goals and priorities, and to help determine the type of positioning technique or devices necessary.

A thorough assessment added to the knowledge of basic positioning will lead to the understanding necessary for the selection of the appropriate solution.

WHEELCHAIR POSITIONING ASSESSMENT FORM

Date:_____   Sex:_____

Name:_____   Age:_____

Diagnosis:_____   Weight:_____

_____   Height:_____

Prognosis:_____

Communication Status:_____

1. Cognitive Function:
   A. Memory:_____

   B. Learning ability:_____

   C. Problem solving:_____

   _____

2. Perceptual Function:
   A. Body awareness:_____
   B. Apraxia:_____
   C. Perseveration:_____
   D. Negligence:_____

3. Sensory Status:
   A. Vision:_____
   B. Hearing:_____
   C. Touch/Pain:_____

4. Transfers:_____
   _____

5. Sitting Balance/Tolerance:_____
   _____

6. Mobility:
   A. Ambulation:_____
   B. Wheelchair mobility:_____

7. Skin Integrity:_____
   _____

8. Use of Arms and Hands:_____
   _____

9. Continence:_____

10. Volition (Personal causation, values, interests):_____
    _____
    _____
    _____
    _____

11. Leisure Interests (Indoor and outdoor activities):_____
    _____
    _____
    _____

12. Living Situation/ Lifestyle:_____
    _____
    _____
    _____

13. Financial Resources:_____
    _____
    _____

Figure 4-1. Wheelchair positioning assessment form.

SEATING STATUS

	Problems (Including range of motion, tone, strength, oedema, deformity)	Corrective Measures
Pelvis		
Hips		
Knees		
Feet		
Trunk control/ Spine		
Head/ Neck		
Shoulders		
Arms/ Hands		

Seating Goals: _____

_____

_____

_____

Signature:_____

Date:_____

5
A Systematic Approach to Positioning

Just as a systematic approach is necessary for basic positioning the same approach is helpful when assessing the problem. The chapters are presented in the following order: buttocks, sacral sitting, lower extremities, trunk, back, head and neck, and upper extremities. Potential problems, special considerations and possible solutions will be discussed for each area.

Every client is unique, as is every positioning problem. There is no "correct" solution to a specific problem. Experimentation will determine the most appropriate positioning device.

For each area of difficulty various solutions are described with general recommendations for their possible use. The proposed solutions may serve as a guide to help create new answers to positioning problems.

Buttocks

Since the wheelchair cushion is the basis for a stable, functional sitting position, a wheelchair should not be prescribed without a cushion. Several factors must be considered when deciding on the most appropriate type of cushion.

Potential Problems

Pressure Sores

Pressure sores or decubitus ulcers are localized areas of cellular necrosis almost always occurring over bony prominences.[13]

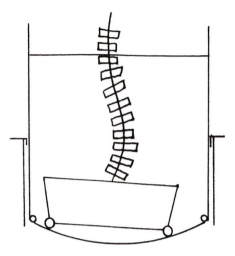

Figure 5-1. Pelvic obliquity.

The two main factors which contribute to pressure sore formation are continuous direct pressure and shearing forces. Problems related to pressure on the tissue vary in degree from redness of the skin on the buttocks, pressure sores, and skin breakdown that results in decreased sitting tolerance.

The parts of the body at risk for pressure sores are the area over the ischial tuberosities, coccyx, sacrum, and the trochanters. Common causes of pressure sores in wheelchairs include:

—Immobility. Inability to shift weight.
—Minimal adipose tissue and/or loss of muscle mass over the buttocks.
—Pelvic obliquity which is caused by the "hammock effect" of the sling seat. It results in increased pressure over one ischial tuberosity and trochanter. This is often accompanied by sideways shearing forces (Refer to Fig. 5-1)
—Pressure sores over the sacrum may be caused by a slumped sitting posture or sacral sitting. The shearing forces, created by the posterior pelvic tilt as the client slides out of the wheelchair, may also contribute to the formation of a sacral pressure sore.

Poor Sitting Posture

—The "hammock effect" of the wheelchair's sling seat is the primary cause of poor sitting posture. The pelvis may tilt to one side (pelvic obliquity), causing the upper body to lean to the side with an accompanying increased lateral curvature of the spine (scoliosis). The "hammock effect" also encourages hip adduction and internal rotation. Sitting balance will be affected due to the poor base of support.
—The "hammock effect" can also encourage sacral sitting, a rounding out of the lower spine, or lumbar-kyphosis, which may become a source of discomfort.

—"Wind swept" deformity—one hip abducted and one hip adducted—causes the legs to appear unequal in length. This complex problem is evidenced by:

- Pelvic obliquity and pelvic rotation. Check the alignment of the anterior superior iliac spines.
- Poor trunk alignment accompanied by discomfort.
- Increased risk of pressure sore over one ischial tuberosity.

Factors contributing to the "wind swept" deformity:

- Muscle imbalance due, for example, to a cerebro-vascular accident or multiple sclerosis.
- Scoliosis or other spinal deformities.
- Short wheelchair seat length, often occurring with clients who are tall or have excessive adipose tissue on the buttocks.

All the potential problems described above lead to one main problem for the client: poor sitting posture in the wheelchair causing discomfort and limited sitting tolerance.

Special Considerations

- When choosing a cushion, consider the following factors:
  —whether the client is continent
  —how easily the cushion can be cleaned
  —whether the cushion requires maintenance
  —the weight of the cushion (if it is necessary to transfer the cushion)
  —cost
  —durability
- A cushion should not be overlayered because this will cause it to lose its property of pressure relief.
- When cushion covers are necessary, two-way stretch material should be used to prevent shearing forces in any direction and to allow conformity with minimal increase in pressure.
- It is advisable to secure the cushion to the wheelchair. Since the cushion can slide forward or back with the client, all four corners require fastening.
- By changing the cushion or the base of support, the height of the seat may alter and require adjustment of the footrests. When footrests are too high, the thighs do not support sufficient body weight, thus increasing the pressure on the ischial tuberosities. If the footrests are too low, the feet do not support body weight and the pressure is increased under the thighs.

Possible Solutions

- Cushions:
  —Polymer Foam
  —Foam cushion with preischial bar
  —KSS Seat Base (Special Health Systems)

    —Roho Cushion (Roho Incorporated)
    —Bard Flotation Cushion (Maddack)
    —Jay Gel Cushion (Jay Medical Ltd.)
  • Level base of support:
    —Plywood board
    —QA2 seat base (QA2 Seating System)
    —SHS Cushion (Special Health Systems)
  • Drop seat base:
    —Wooden drop seat
    —QA2 drop seat base (QA2 Seating System)
    —SHS Fiberglass low seat (Special Health Systems)
  • Long seat base.

Cushions

According to several studies, no type of cushion is superior at relieving pressure for all clients.[14, 15, 16] The ideal cushion would distribute pressure evenly over the largest skin area. All cushions available to date have positive and negative features. To determine the most appropriate type of cushion, an assessment is necessary to meet individual needs and ensure good posture and pressure relief. The assessment should include:

    —diagnosis
    —number of hours spent in the wheelchair daily
    —urinary control
    —history of skin breakdown
    —body build
    —postural problems
    —climate

The following is a description of six cushions. They can be divided into three categories.

    —Polymer foam
    —Air-filled
    —Flotation (gel or water filled)

Polymer Foam

Polymer foam cushion is the standard wheelchair cushion. Polymer foam is lightweight, breathable, and inexpensive. It is easily modified to the needs of the individual client by cutting, wedging or gluing.

Foam cushions are not washable and they wear out faster than other types of cushion. As they are lightweight, it may be necessary to tie the cushions to the wheelchair to prevent them from sliding forward. A standard wheelchair cushion is made of 7.5 cm. (3 in.) medium density foam.

Foam Cushion With Preischial Bar

A foam cushion with preischial bar can be used for clients who develop redness over the posterior aspect of the buttocks. Pressure is transferred from

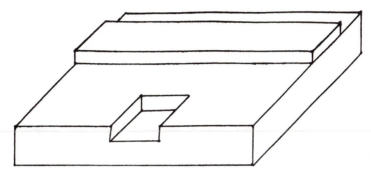

Figure 5-2. Foam cushion with preischial bar.

the sacral, coccygeal, and ischial areas to the back of the well-padded thighs. A hole is made at the back of the cushion to decrease the pressure over the coccygeal region.

Construction:

1. A cushion is cut to fit the size of the wheelchair seat out of 7.5 cm. (3 in.) medium density foam.
2. A piece of medium density foam 2.5 cm. (1 in.) high, 10 cm. (4 in.) wide, with the same width as the cushion, is glued at 5 cm. (2 in.) from the front end.
3. A space 6 cm. (2.5 in.) wide, 6 cm. (2.5 in.) long, and 2.5 cm. (1 in.) deep is cut in the middle at the back. (Refer to Fig. 5-2)
4. The cover is made of a durable and stretchable fabric. Ties are sewn at the back to attach the cushion to the wheelchair.

KSS Seat Base (Special Health Systems)

The KSS seat base is a positioning cushion made of foam on a solid plywood base.

The cushion has an anterior wedge to prevent pelvic tilting or sliding. It also has a firm preischial bar that transfers pressure from the sacral, coccygeal, and ischial region to the back of the well-padded thighs.

Leg channels provide a balanced neutral leg position and prevent rotation at the hips.

To Assemble:

The KSS seat base is made of 5 cm. (2 in.) medium density foam and a layer of 2.5 cm. (1 in.) comfort foam.

The preischial bar is made of 2.5 cm. (1 in.) medium density foam. The KSS seat base is suspended on the wheelchair frame with four stainless steel snap-on suspension hooks after the sling seat is removed.

The cushion has a stretch terry cover over a water resistent neoprene shell.

The KSS seat base can be fitted to most types of standard adult wheelchair or reclining wheelchair. It is available in 2 standard sizes: 41 cm. (16 in.) and 46 cm. (18 in.) wide.

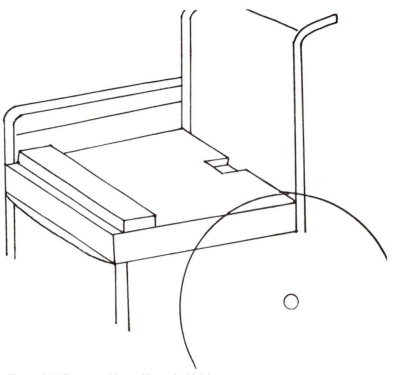

Figure 5-3. Foam cushion with preischial bar.

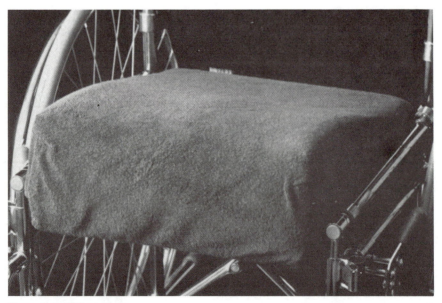

Figure 5-4. KSS seat base.

Roho Cushion (Roho, Inc.)

The High Profile Roho cushion remains the cushion of choice in the preventing and/or healing of decubitus ulcers in long-term or high-risk sitting.

The Roho cushion is an air-filled type cushion. It is not a cushion for sitting "on" but rather a cushion for sitting "in". The immersion assures maximum skin contact and conformity, and maintains good pelvic stability. It is preferable to use the cushion without a cover to achieve the lowest amount of skin pressure.

The Roho cushion does not provide stability, and therefore is not recommended for clients who slide forward in their wheelchair or who have a poor sitting position due to extension contractures of the hips.

This cushion is lightweight, easy to clean and easy to transfer. The air pressure should be checked regularly to assure correct pressure and to maximize sitting stability.

The High Profile Roho cushion is available in two standard sizes: regular adult 38 x 43 x 10 cm. (15 x 17 x 4 in.) and narrow adult 38 x 38 x 10 cm. (15 x 15 x 4 in.)

To Assemble:

To use a Roho cushion:

1. Inflate the cushion until the middle of the cushion begins to arch slightly.
2. Sit the client on the inflated cushion.
3. Insert one hand under the buttocks, palm upward, with finger tips touching one ischial tuberosity.
4. Deflate the cushion until the clearance between the bony prominence and the base of the cushion is one finger's thickness (1.2 cm. or 0.5 in.)

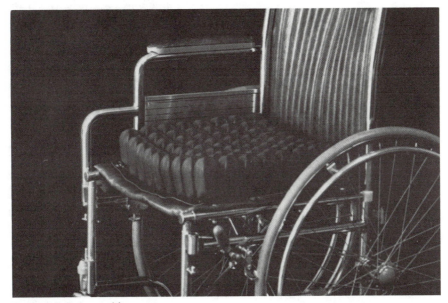

Figure 5-5. Roho cushion.

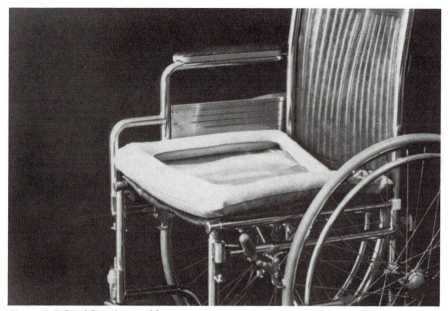

Figure 5-6. Bard flotation cushion.

Bard Flotation Cushion (Maddack)

The Bard flotation cushion is recommended for clients who are at risk for pressure sores and who require stabilization of the pelvis.

The cushion comes in two parts: a water-filled cushion and an air frame. The air frame provides good pelvic and trunk stability. The water-filled cushion assures even pressure distribution. While easy to clean, it may be too heavy for clients who need to transfer the cushion independently.

To Assemble:

The Bard flotation cushion is available in one size 46 x 41 cm. (18 x 16 in.)

Since the cushion is filled with water, some clients may find it pleasantly cool while others may find it cold. A sheet of 0.5 cm. (3/16 in.) thick, low-temperature, closed-cell foam, such as plastazote, can be used to insulate the water filled cushion. To maximize the effectiveness of the cushion, the cover used should be a durable and stretchable fabric.

Jay Gel Cushion (Jay Medical, Ltd.)

The Jay gel flotation cushion is designed to stabilize the pelvis, level the hips, and provide trunk stability. It also promotes a neutral leg position.

The Jay gel cushion is recommended for clients who need postural support and who are at high risk for skin problems from sitting in the wheelchair for long periods of time.

The Jay gel cushion comes in two parts: a urethane contoured foam base

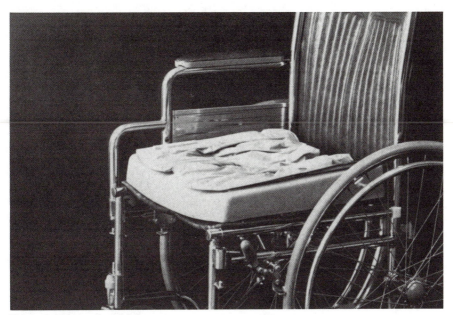

Figure 5-7. Jay gel cushion.

and a Flolite pad. The pad is segmented to prevent bottoming out. The foam base has a slight backward angle to prevent the client from sliding forward. It also has a nonskid bottom to prevent the cushion from sliding in the wheelchair. The Jay gel cushion is easy to clean and needs to be stored flat.

To Assemble:

The Jay gel cushion is available in five different sizes: regular adult, narrow adult, regular adult long, narrow adult long, and junior. The regular adult long and the narrow adult long are used mainly with a reclining wheelchair.

Overfilled pads or fluid supplement pads can be ordered for thin clients to prevent bottoming out of the cushion. Single, double or triple overfilled pads are available. The single overfilled pad is frequently used. An overfilled pad is needed if at least 0.6 cm. (0.25 in.) of fluid remains where the ischials and coccyx are positioned after the client has sat on the cushion for two minutes.

Level Base of Support

A level base of support is necessary to counteract the "hammock effect" of the sling seat. It prevents pelvic obliquity, thus helping to distribute the pressure evenly under both buttocks, and can also assist in preventing upper body leaning. A level base of support promotes neutral rotation at the hips and neutral leg position.

The following three methods provide a level base of support.

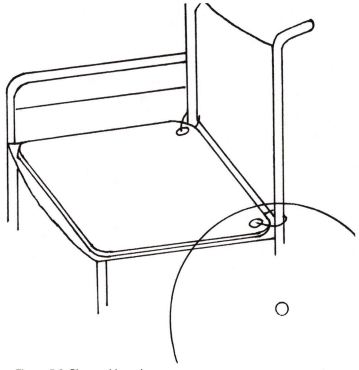

Figure 5-8. Plywood board.

Plywood Board

Construction:

1. A board of 1 cm. (3/8 in.) plywood is cut to fit the size of the wheelchair seat. The corners are rounded.
2. The board is placed on top of the sling seat and must be supported on the two seat rails.
3. Two holes are drilled in the back corners of the board and ties are used to secure the board to the back frame of the wheelchair.
4. A cushion is then placed on the plywood and fixed with velcro to prevent sliding forward or backward. The foam and cover can be stapled to the plywood board.

QA2 Seat Base (QA2 Seating System)

The QA2 seat base is made of strong ABS thermal plastic. The seat base inserts on the wheelchair seat rails with no modification to the wheelchair.

The QA2 seat base can be fitted to most types of standard adult wheelchairs and reclining wheelchairs with widths ranging from 36 cm. (14 in.) to 51 cm. (20 in.) with varying seat depths.

QA2 flat or wedge cushions are available and are secured to the seat base with velcro. The wedge cushion is 7.5 cm. (3 in.) thick at the front and 5 cm.

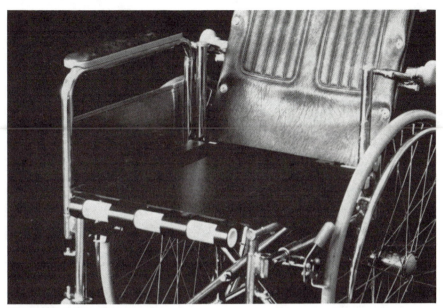

Figure 5-9. QA2 seat base.

(2 in.) thick at the back. Cushions are made of medium density foam with a water resistant Ultraskin cover.

SHS Cushion (Special Health Systems)

The SHS cushion fits the contour of the sling seat and provides a level sitting surface. There are two types of SHS cushions: one for standard seating requirements and one for sensitive seating requirements. The SHS cushion comes in standard or wedge (2.5 cm. or 1 in. lower at the back).

Standard SHS cushions are made of 5 cm. (2 in.) or 2.5 cm. (1 in.) medium density foam and 2.5 cm. (1 in.) comfort foam. Cushions for sensitive seating requirements have an extra 2.5 cm. (1 in.) contouring foam.

The cushions are covered with a durable and waterproof stretch neoprene cover. An outer covering is available in stretch terry cloth.

The SHS cushions are 43.5 x 43.5 cm. (17 x 17 in.) to fit narrow and regular adult wheelchair sling seats.

Drop Seat Base

A drop seat base can be used with any type of cushion to prevent buildup of the height of the seat, and to provide a level base of support.

Various problems may be created by a seat which is too high:

—Mobilization of the wheelchair with the lower extremities becomes difficult or impossible.
—Transferring may become hazardous.
—Armrests and back height may be too low, thus affecting trunk stability.

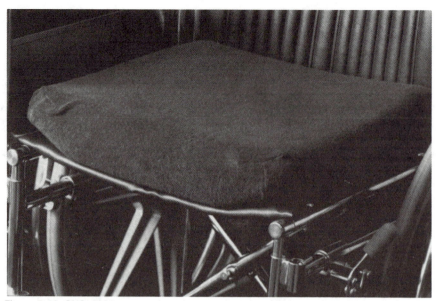

Figure 5-10. SHS cushion.

—Environmental difficulties, such as being unable to get the knees under a table, often occur.

Wooden Drop Seat

The wooden drop seat lowers the seating surface by 5 cm. (2 in.).

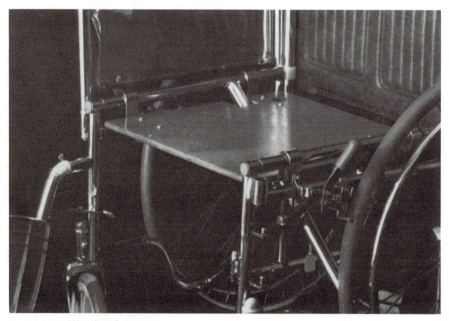

Figure 5-11. Wooden drop seat.

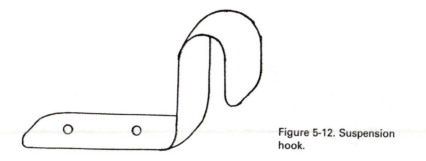

Figure 5-12. Suspension hook.

Construction:

The wooden drop seat is made of 1 cm. (3/8 in.) plywood and four stainless steel suspension hooks (wheelchair brackets, IDC Tectonics Ltd.). For a 46 cm. (18 in.) wide wheelchair with the sling seat removed:

1. Cut a piece of plywood 40 cm. (15.75 in.) long and 38.5 cm. (15 in.) wide.
2. Two spaces 3 cm. (1.25 in.) wide and 6 cm. (2.5 in.) long are cut so the board will fit over the cross bars (Refer to Fig. 5-11).
   —The four suspension hooks are fixed to the board with bolts.
   —It is advisable to tie the drop seat to the wheelchair, as the seat may tilt forward if the client slides forward in the wheelchair.

QA2 Drop Seat Base (QA2 Seating System)

The QA2 drop seat base can be fitted to most types of standard adult wheelchairs and reclining wheelchairs with widths from 36 cm. (14 in.) to 46 cm. (18 in.)

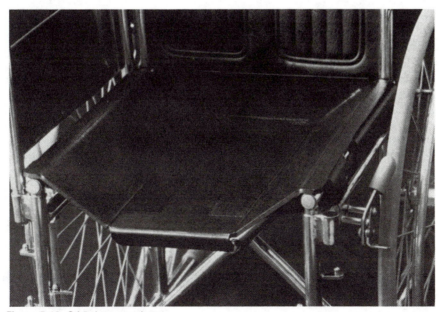

Figure 5-13. QA2 drop seat base.

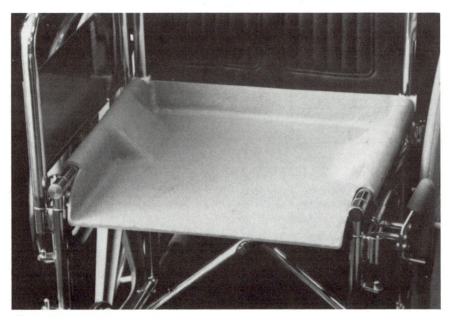

Figure 5-14. SHS Fiberglass low seat.

The molded seat base inserts onto the wheelchair seat rails with the sling seat removed. The drop seat base is secured to the wheelchair with two velcro straps located under the seat base. It lowers the height of the seat by 6.5 cm. (2.5 in.)

The drop seat base can be fitted with a QA2 flat cushion or a wedge cushion. The cushion is fixed to the drop seat base with velcro. It is made of medium density foam with a water resistant Ultraskin cover.

SHS Fiberglass Low Seat (Special Health Systems)

The SHS fiberglass low seat can be fitted to most types of standard adult wheelchairs and reclining wheelchairs. It is available in one standard size: 46 cm. (18 in.) wide.

The molded fiberglass seat inserts onto the wheelchair seat rails with the sling seat removed. It lowers the seating surface by 6.5 cm. (2.5 in.).

A compatible SHS low seat cushion made of 5 cm. (2 in.) medium density foam with a neoprene shell and a stretch terry cover can be used with the fiberglass low seat.

Long Seat Base

When a longer seat base is required, for example with clients who have a "wind swept" deformity due to a short seat length, a customized wheelchair can be ordered.

Another solution is to make an extra long wooden drop seat that is securely fastened in all four corners of the wheelchair frame. Refer to Buttocks, Wooden Drop Seat. The length of the seat will vary according to the client's measurements and requirements.

Sacral Sitting—The Slider

Since the pelvis is the foundation on which the trunk is balanced, pelvic stability is the prerequisite to performing functional activities with the upper extremities, lower extremities, and head.

The "slider" slips forward in the wheelchair, often ending up with the buttocks on the front of the seat, the weight on the sacrum, the feet out on the floor in front of the footrests, and the shoulders halfway down the back of the wheelchair. In this position, the client will usually have back pain and be unable to mobilize the wheelchair. This position is called sacral sitting.

The solution to the problem varys according to the cause. Therefore, a good assessment is essential.

Potential Problems

Various factors can cause a client to slide in the wheelchair:

- Hypertonicity of the extensor muscles of the lower extremities and trunk may result in difficulty achieving and/or maintaining hip and knee flexion.
- Extension contractures at the hips limit the ability to attain the sitting position. This may be combined with extension contractures of the knees and ankles, in which case good positioning of the legs is essential.
- With hypotonicity or weakness of the trunk and muscles of the lower extremities, the client may be unable to stop sliding down in the wheelchair.
- Occasionally, a client may slide down in the wheelchair in order to get attention.
- Medical problems that may be contributing to discomfort in the sitting position should be considered. Some clients may have difficulty communicating exactly why they are restless. For example, a client with back pain may slide forward in the wheelchair to ease the pain, but may be unable to push himself or herself back up in the wheelchair.
- The client may slide forward to mobilize the wheelchair with the lower extremities. To provide freedom of movement for the lower extremities, the patient moves the buttock forward in the wheelchair.

Special Considerations

- Is the seat depth correct? If the seat is too short or too long, a custom-made wheelchair with an appropriate seat length may be part of the solution to sliding.
- Roho cushion is usually inappropriate for a client who has a tendency to slide, particularly those who have increased extensor tone or extension contractures of the hips. The Roho cushion does not provide stability on its own.
- Nylon cushion covers should be avoided. Nylon reduces friction and facilitates movement in the wheelchair, but it may also facilitate sliding.
- Are the feet well supported? To stabilize the client in the wheelchair, the feet must be comfortably positioned and flat on the footrest. It is very

difficult for the client to push back and sit upright if the feet are not well supported.

- Exercise caution when using restraints in a wheelchair, especially with chest-type restraints. These rarely prevent sliding and may even encourage sliding as the client becomes restless in the wheelchair. Any restraint will interfere with the client's freedom of movement. Careful thought and assessment is necessary when considering this alternative.
- A wedge cushion is frequently used to prevent sliding, but this will change the seat height. This may interfere with the client's ability to mobilize the wheelchair with the lower extremities and to transfer from the wheelchair. The height of the footrests may need to be adjusted to the changed seat height.
- If a client tends to slide on the seat, shearing is generated in the tissue. Caregivers must be alert for skin breakdown over the buttocks in the sacral sitter.

Possible Solutions

- Wedge foam cushion
- Wedge board with foam cushion
- Foam cushion with preischial bar
- Bard flotation cushion (Maddack)
- Forty-five degree lapbelt (Special Health Systems)
- Drop seat with wedge cushion
  —Wooden drop seat
  —Postura Inclinable Seat (Everest and Jennings)
  —QA2 drop seat base with wedge cushion (QA2 Seating System)
  —KSS seat base (Special Health Systems)

Wedge Foam Cushion

A wedge foam cushion is a simple solution for mild problems of sacral sitting. It will help to maintain position of the hips as far back on the seat as possible.

A wedge cushion can be used with any type of adult wheelchair, but is often used with a reclining wheelchair to maintain hip flexion at about 100 degrees.

The cushion should be tied to the back frame of the wheelchair to prevent it from sliding forward with the client. The footrest height should be adjusted to accommodate the increased seat height caused by the wedge cushion.

To avoid increasing the seat height, a drop seat can be fitted; this will be especially useful if the client is mobilizing the wheelchair with the lower extremities.

Construction:

1. A wedge cushion is cut out of medium density foam to fit the size of the wheelchair seat.
2. To maintain 100 degrees of hip flexion, a thickness of 5 cm. (2 in.) at the back and 10 to 15 cm. (4 to 6 in.) at the front is used.

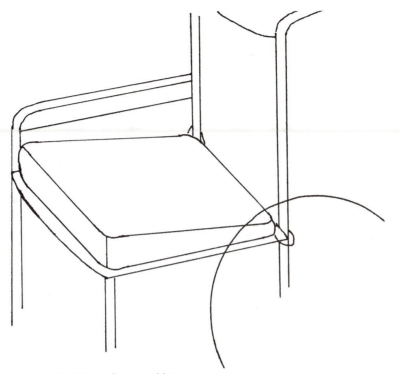

Figure 5-15. Wedge foam cushion.

3. The cushion is covered with a durable and stretchable fabric. Slippery fabric such as nylon should be avoided.
4. Ties are sewn at the back of the cover to secure the cushion to the wheelchair frame.

Wedge Board With Foam Cushion

The wedge board with foam cushion is recommended to prevent mild to moderate problems of sacral sitting and sliding. The addition of the board will also provide a more firm sitting surface to prevent pelvic obliquity.

If positioning a client in a reclining wheelchair, a wedge board with foam cushion can be used to maintain hip flexion at about 100 degrees.

The wedge board should be tied to the back frame of the wheelchair to prevent it from sliding forward with the client.

The height of the footrests should be adjusted to accommodate the increased seat height caused by the wedge.

Construction:

The board is made of 0.6 cm. (0.25 in.) plywood and 1.2 cm. (1 in.) plywood.

1. Cut two pieces of 0.6 cm. (0.25 in.) plywood the same width and depth as the wheelchair seat.
2. Cut one piece of the 1.2 cm. (1 in.) plywood the width of the wheelchair

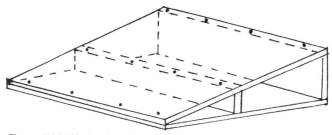

Figure 5-16. Wedge board.

seat. The height depends on the height required at the front of the wedge, which is usually 3 cm. (1.25 in.) high for a wedge board with cushion of 10 cm. (4 in.) high. Cut another length 2 cm. (1.75 in.) high.

3. The wedge board is assembled according to Fig.5-16. All the pieces are glued and nailed together.
4. The wedge board is varnished for cleanliness.
5. A cushion is cut out of 5 cm. (2 in.) medium density foam to fit the size of the wedge board.
6. The cover is made with a durable and stretchable fabric. The cover and foam cushion are stapled to the wedge board to prevent the cushion from sliding forward.

Foam Cushion With Preischial Bar

The foam cushion with preischial bar is used for mild problems of sacral sitting and to counteract forward sliding in the wheelchair, as it transfers some of the weight from the sacrum to the thighs. It can be used with any standard adult wheelchair or reclining wheelchair.

After the cushion is fitted, footrest height may need to be adjusted to the increased seat height. The cushion should be attached to the back of the wheelchair frame to prevent it from sliding forward with the client.

Construction:

To make a foam cushion with a preischial bar, refer to Buttocks, Foam Cushion With Preischial Bar.

Bard Flotation Cushion (Maddack)

The Bard flotation cushion is used to prevent sacral sitting and sliding forward in the wheelchair. It is effective in preventing sliding when 100 degrees of hip flexion cannot be achieved due to mild extension contractures. The air-filled frame of this water cushion provides stability to the pelvis. If extension contractures are severe, other approaches or adaptations may be considered.

The Bard Flotation cushion does not slide or move in the wheelchair due to its weight and therefore can prevent sliding of clients who have increased extensor tone or extensor spasm in the lower extremities or the whole body.

Any type of adult wheelchair 46 cm. (18 in.) wide can be fitted with this cushion. When fitting a Bard flotation cushion, the footrest height will need to be adjusted to the increased seat height.

It is not advisable to use the Bard flotation cushion with very heavy clients.

To Assemble:

Refer to Buttocks, Bard Flotation Cushion.

Forty-Five Degree Lap Belt (Special Health Systems)

The 45 degree angle lap belt is used to prevent the pelvis from tilting and sliding forward.

The lap belt will restrain the client from transferring independently or repositioning in the wheelchair and so it should be used only if sacral sitting and sliding can not be prevented by positioning with a cushion.

An appropriate cushion (one of the types recommended for sacral sitting) should be used in conjunction with the lap belt. A 45 degree angle lap belt can be fitted to any type of adult wheelchair.

To Assemble:

The SHS 45 degree angle lap belt is made of 5 cm (2 in.) wide nylon webbing with a light weight plastic buckle at the front.

It is secured with the back screws on the seat rails of the wheelchair. The lap belt is positioned over the iliac crest (hip bone) at a 45 degree angle. It should fit snugly but comfortably.

Other types of seat belt used should be positioned on the wheelchair in the same way.

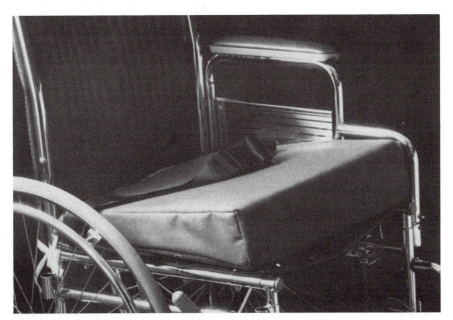

Figure 5-17. Forty-five degree lap belt.

Drop Seat With Wedge Cushion

A drop seat with wedge cushion is used for the same reason as a wedge foam cushion: to prevent sacral sitting and sliding forward and out of the wheelchair.

The purpose of the drop seat is to prevent building up of the seat height. This is especially important for clients who mobilize the wheelchair with the lower extremities.

A seat which is too high may cause environmental difficulties, such as a client being unable to get knees under a table. With a high seat the armrest and back height may be too low to provide adequate support causing poor posture and trunk instability.

Wooden Drop Seat

The wooden drop seat lowers the height of the seat by 5 cm. (2 in.). It can be used in conjunction with any type of wedge cushion. For construction, refer to Buttocks, Wooden Drop Seat.

Postura Inclinable Seat (Everest and Jennings)

The Postura inclinable seat can be fitted to most Everest and Jennings standard adult wheelchairs with detachable armrests, and semi-reclining and fully-reclining wheelchairs. It is available in two adult sizes: adult 46 cm. (18 in.) and narrow adult 41 cm. (16 in.). When considering using the Postura inclinable seat with any type of wheelchair other than Everest and Jennings, consult a local dealer for feasibility.

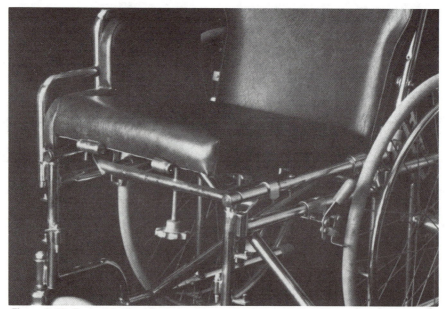

Figure 5-18. Postura inclinable seat.

To Assemble:

The sling seat is removed and the inclinable seat is mounted on the wheelchair seat rails with suspension hooks. The seat provides elevation up to 15 cm. (6 in.). A bolt and handle under the seat adjusts the angle of inclination.

QA2 Drop Seat Base With Wedge Cushion (QA2 Seating System)

The QA2 drop seat base with wedge cushion is available in a wide selection of sizes to fit most types of adult wheelchairs, ranging from 36 cm. (14 in.) to 46 cm. (18 in.) wide. It lowers the height of the seat by 6.5 cm. (2.5 in.).

The ABS plastic molded seat base is inserted onto the wheelchair seat rails with the sling seat removed. The drop seat base is secured to the wheelchair with two velcro straps situated under the seat base.

The wedge cushion is 8 cm. (3 in.) thick at the front and 5 cm. (2 in.) thick at the back. It is made of medium density foam with a water resistant Ultraskin cover. The cushion is fixed to the seat base with velcro. To increase effectiveness, a 45 degree lap belt can be used in conjunction with the drop seat base.

To Assemble:

Refer to Buttocks, QA2 Drop Seat Base.

KSS Seat Base (Special Health Systems)

The KSS seat base is a foam cushion on a solid plywood base.

The cushion has an anterior wedge to prevent pelvic tilting and sliding. It includes a firm preischial bar that transfers some of the weight from the sacral, coccygeal and ischial region to the back of the well padded thighs. The cushion has leg channels to provide a balanced neutral leg position and neutral rotation at the hips.

The sling seat is first removed and the seat base is then secured with four stainless steel snap on suspension hooks onto the wheelchair seat rails.

To Assemble:

Refer to Buttocks, KSS Seat Base.

Lower Extremities

The reasons for intervention in the positioning of the lower extremities varies considerably, since individuals with the same physical disability may present with different problems.

Trunk stability and balance are affected by the position of the lower extremities.

Potential Problems

- One or both feet fall off the footrest/legrest. They may fall behind, to the side, or in front of the footrest. The feet may be injured by the front casters or they may drag on the floor.

This may be due to flaccidity, spasticity, or weakness (slight or severe) of one or both lower extremities.

The client may be unable to alert the caregiver, unable to independently lift the foot back onto the footrest, or be unaware that the foot is on the floor because of a lack of awareness of body position or impaired sensitivity.

- Lack of comfortable support for the foot caused by a foot plate which is too low.
- Pain or discomfort of the above- or below-knee amputee, usually caused by the lack of support for an amputated extremity. The end of the stump requires protection when the client is mobilizing in a wheelchair. For the below-knee amputee, contractures of the knee must be prevented if the client wears a prosthesis.
- Oedema. A swelling which is present in the ankle may extend up the calf.
- Injury of the lower extremities through uncontrolled movements, such as spasms, or from a lack of awareness of body position.
- An open sore on the lateral aspect of the knee caused by pressure against the raised pivot point of the elevating legrest.
- Poor sitting balance caused by adductor spasticity which results in trunk leaning to one side or pressure sores on the medial aspect of the knees.
- "Wind swept" deformity—one hip abducted and one hip adducted— causes the legs to appear unequal in length. Since this is a complex problem, various factors—rotation of the pelvis, pelvic obliquity, muscle imbalance and/or short wheelchair seat length—may cause this deformity. Refer to Buttocks, Potential Problems, "Wind Swept" Deformity.
- Plantar flexion deformity resulting in difficulty positioning the foot on the foot plate.

Special Considerations

- Transfer modality
  The method used to transfer the client from the wheelchair to the bed will affect the choice of a positioning device. A legrest cradle, for example, may prevent the client's legs from falling off the footrests, but standing pivot transfers will become difficult for the client and the caregiver.
- Changing the center of gravity of a wheelchair by fully elevating both legrests may be dangerous. A standard frame wheelchair is not designed to accommodate the extra weight at the front, especially if the client is tall and/or heavy. The wheelchair may easily tip forward. This can be prevented by adding anti-tipping weights at the back of the wheelchair or by using a reclining wheelchair.

Possible Solutions

- Elevating blocks on foot plates
- Knee protector for elevating legrests
- Heel strap

- Legrest panel:
  - —Fabric legrest panel
  - —Legrest panel—one piece Hook-on Leatherette (Everest and Jennings).
- Foot support:
  - —Wooden foot support
  - —SHS Foot support kit (Special Health Systems)
- Board support on legrests:
  - —Legrest board
  - —Leg and footrest board
- Padded wooden legrest
- Postura legrest cradle (Everest and Jennings)
- Above knee amputee cushion
- Figure "8" foot strap
- Ankle Positioning Aids:
  - —Ankle positioning blocks
  - —Foot plates with adjustable angle setting (Everest and Jennings)
- Knee abductor

Elevating Blocks on Foot Plates

If the foot plates are raised to their shortest position and the clients feet still are not supported on the foot plates, a comfortable support can be provided through the use of elevating blocks.

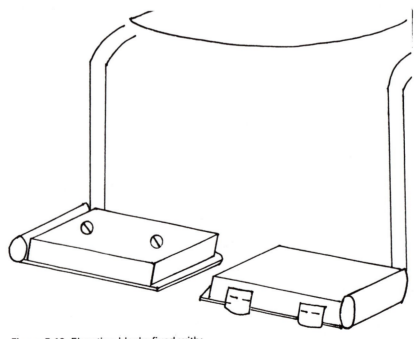

Figure 5-19. Elevating blocks fixed with:
   1. Bolts
   2. Wide elastic strap.

Construction:

1. Elevating blocks are made of 5 cm. (2 in.) by 15 cm. (6 in.) lumber cut to fit the size of the foot plate.
2. To confirm the height of the foot plate slip two fingers under the thigh to a depth of approximately 3.75 to 5 cm. (1.5 to 2 in.)
3. Secure the block to the foot plate with two bolts. The block and the foot plate are drilled and the nut is screwed under the foot plate.
4. Another method of securing the block to the foot plate is with an elastic strap. A 5 cm. (2 in.) wide strip of elastic is stapled to the two sides of the block and loops under the foot plate. The first method of securing the block is preferable, as it is a more permanent solution.

Knee Protector for Elevating Legrests

When using elevating legrests the lateral aspect of the knee may press against the raised pivot point of the legrest.

This area is at risk for the development of a pressure sore and is often a source of discomfort.

Construction:

1. The knee protector is made of 1.2 cm. (0.5 in.) low-temperature, closed-cell foam, such as plastazote, which is cut as shown in Fig. 5-20.
2. Mold the plastazote around the raised pivot point of the hinge. To position, refer to Fig. 5-20; "A" is the top section and "C" is the bottom section. Bend at "B" over the pivot point.
3. The knee protector is held in place with 2.5 cm. (1 in.) wide velcro straps.

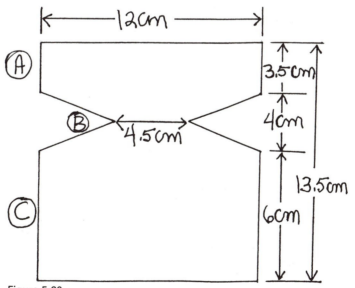

Figure 5-20.

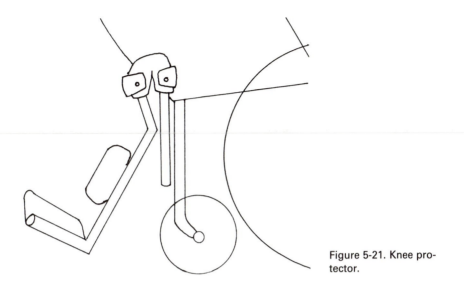

Figure 5-21. Knee pro-
tector.

Heel Straps

The heel strap is used to prevent the feet from falling off the back of the footrests.

When increased tone in the flexor muscles of the lower extremities is the cause of this problem, the heel strap is not recommended because the feet will probably still rise over the heel strap and get caught behind the footrest.

Construction:

1. The heel strap is made of a strong durable material, such as leather or webbing, approximately 7.5 to 10 cm. (3 to 4 in.) wide. If necessary, two lengths of webbing can be sewn together.
2. The strap is long enough to wrap around the footrest and overlap by 10 to 12.5 cm. (4 to 5 in.). The heel strap is secured using velcro.

Legrest Panel

The legrest panel prevents the lower extremities from falling between and behind the footrests.

It is recommended for use with clients who have increased tone in the flexor muscles of the lower extremities or who have weakness or lack of awareness of the lower extremities.

The legrest panel can be used with footrests or with elevating legrests.

Construction:

Fabric Legrest Panel

Use a durable material such as leatherette or denim.

1. To fit a 41 cm. or 46 cm. (16 or 18 in.) wide adult wheelchair, cut a piece of material 28 cm. (11 in.) long and 43 cm. (17 in.) wide.
2. Four lengths of 5 cm. (2 in.) wide velcro are sewn, one in each corner,

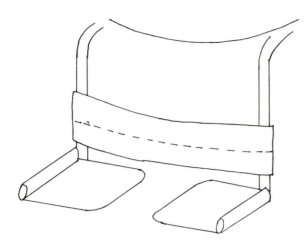

Figure 5-22. Heel strap.

to attach the legrest panel to the footrest. A 7 cm. (2.5 in.) strip of hook velcro is sewn on the corner of the panel with the adjoining 15 cm. (6 in.) strip of loop velcro.

Legrest Panel—One piece hook-on leatherette (Everest and Jennings)

This leatherette legrest panel is useful with elevating legrests or footrests. It easily attaches to the legrests with four metal hooks.

It is not appropriate for clients who have severe spasticity of the flexor muscles of the lower extremities because the metal hooks may be stretched by the constant leg pressure against the panel. Standard widths available are 41 cm. (16 in.) and 46 cm. (18 in.).

Foot Support

The foot support prevents the feet from falling between or behind the foot plates and is used with clients who have flaccidity, weakness or mild increase

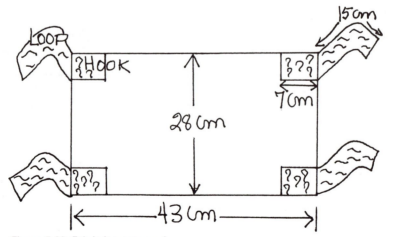

Figure 5-23. Fabric legrest panel.

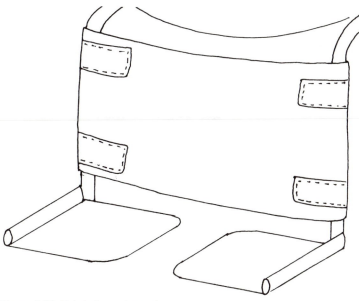

Figure 5-24. Fabric legrest panel.

in extensor tone of one or both lower extremities. It is also useful in preventing foot injury for clients who have poor body awareness.

It provides good support for the whole length of the foot. The foot support can be mounted on footrests or elevating legrests. It is secured to only one foot plate which permits it to swing away with the footrest for ease of transfer.

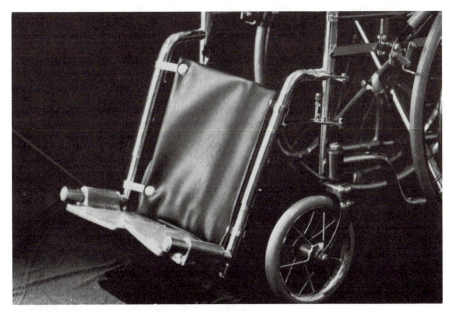

Figure 5-25. Everest and Jennings legrest panel.

Construction:

Wooden Foot Support
   Use 0.6 cm. (0.25 in.) plywood.

   1. To fit a 46 cm. (18 in.) wide adult wheelchair, cut the following pieces:

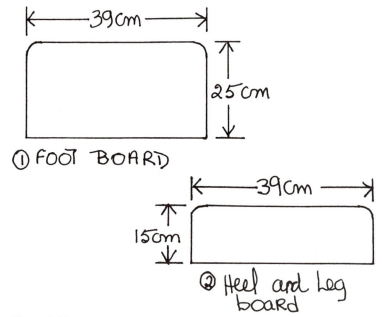

Figure 5-26.

   2. Pieces 1 and 2 are fixed together at 90 degrees with two 5 cm. (2 in.) long corner braces and bolts.
   3. Two holes are drilled in one side of the foot board to align with two holes drilled in one side of the foot plate.

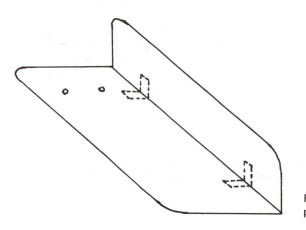

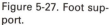
Figure 5-27. Foot support.

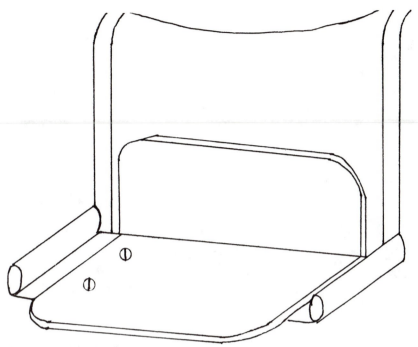

Figure 5-28. Wooden foot support.

4. The wooden foot support can be either varnished or padded with 2.5 cm. (1 in.) low density foam covered with a durable fabric, such as denim.
5. The wooden foot support is secured to one foot plate with two bolts.

SHS Foot Support Kit (Special Health Systems)

The foot support kit is made of strong thermoplastic material.

It is mounted on the right foot plate extending across the left foot plate to provide support for both feet.

The foot support swings away with the footrest for ease of transfer. It can be fitted to 41 cm. (16 in.) or 46 cm. (18 in.) wide wheelchairs.

Board Support on Legrests

The board support is intended to provide support to the lower extremities and prevent them from falling between or behind elevating legrests. This support can also be used with clients who have a below knee amputation.

A foot board can be added to provide support to the feet.

It is convenient for use with clients who transfer with a mechanical lift, as the board would not have to be removed during transfer.

Construction:

Legrest Board

Use 0.5 cm. (0.25 in.) plywood.

1. To determine the width of the board required, measure the distance

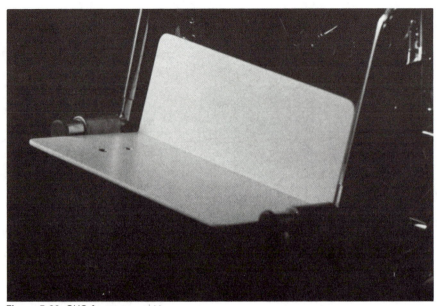

Figure 5-29. SHS foot support kit.

between the legrests within the posts. For example, for a 46 cm. (18 in.) wide adult wheelchair use a board 39 cm. (15.5 in.) wide.

2. The length of the legrest board depends on the client's leg length. Measure from just below the raised pivot point on the legrest to the bottom of the clients calf.

3. The corners of the board are rounded and two holes 2 cm. (0.75 in.) diameter are drilled in the upper corners.

4. The board is padded with 2.5 cm. (1 in.) low density foam and covered with a soft but durable fabric. The cover is stapled to the back of the board.

5. Two 2.5 cm. (1 in.) wide velcro straps secured to the holes attach the legrest board to the wheelchair.

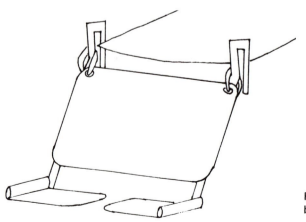

Figure 5-30. Legrest board.

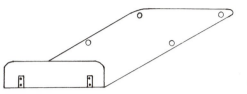

Figure 5-31. Leg and footrest board.

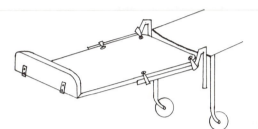

Figure 5-32. Leg and footrest board.

Leg and Footrest Board

Use 0.5 cm. (0.25 in.) plywood.

1. To determine the width of the board, measure the distance between the legrests within the posts. For example, a 46 cm. (18 in.) wide adult wheelchair requires a board 39 cm. (15.5 in.) wide.
2. The length of the board depends on the clients leg length. Measure from just below the raised pivot point on the legrest to the client's heel with the ankle at 90 degrees, or to the toes if the client has a drop foot. Add 2.5 cm. (1 in.) to that measurement.
3. The top two corners of the board are rounded. Four holes 2 cm. (0.75 in.) dia. are drilled; two in the upper corners and one on each side halfway down the board. (Refer to Fig. 5-31).
4. The foot board is cut the same width as the leg board. The height of the board is determined by adding 5 cm. (2 in.) to the length of the client's foot. The two top corners are rounded. (Refer to Fig. 5-31)
5. The leg board and foot board are secured together at 90 degrees using two corner braces 5 cm. (2 in.) long and 2 cm. (0.75 in.) long bolts.
6. The board is padded with a 2.5 cm. (1 in.) low density foam and covered with a soft, durable fabric. The cover is stapled to the back of the board.
7. Four 2.5 cm. (1 in.) velcro straps attach through the holes to secure the board to the legrests. The wheelchair foot plates can be removed if necessary.

Padded Wooden Legrest

The padded wooden legrest provides additional protection and support for one lower extremity on an elevating legrest.

It prevents the leg from falling off the elevating legrest and provides a larger area of support.

The padded wooden legrest can be fitted to any type of elevating legrest.

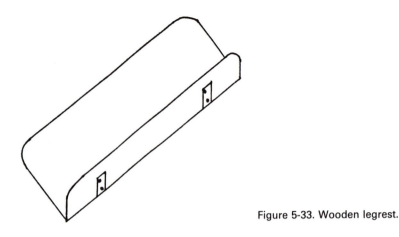

Figure 5-33. Wooden legrest.

It does not interfere with the client's ability to transfer, as it is attached to the mounting bracket of the standard legrest panel and can be swung away.

Construction:
Use a 1 cm. (3/8 in.) plywood.

1. Cut two pieces of plywood:
   —35 cm. (14 in.) long by 7.5 cm. (3 in.) wide
   —35 cm. (14 in.) long by 18 cm. (7 in.) wide
   Round the corners (Refer to Fig. 5-33)

2. The pieces are joined at a right angle with two 4 cm. (1.5 in.) long corner braces and bolts.

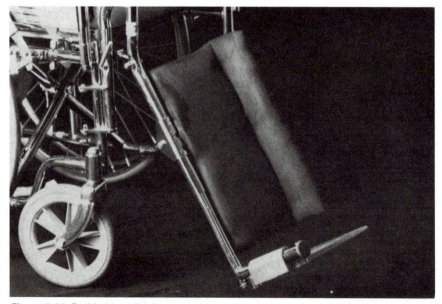

Figure 5-34. Padded wooden legrest.

3. The original legrest panel is removed from the elevating legrest and the wooden legrest is secured to the mounting bracket with bolts.
4. The wooden legrest is padded with 2.5 cm. (1 in.) low density foam.
5. It can be covered with any soft, durable fabric. The cover is stapled to the padded wooden legrest.

Postura Legrest Cradle (Everest and Jennings)

The Postura legrest cradle is used for more severe positioning problems of both lower extremities.

If the lower extremities tend to fall off standard elevating legrests, the legrest cradle can be used to provide extra support and to protect the leg from injury.

The Postura legrest cradle can be fitted to most Everest and Jennings standard adult wheelchair or semi-reclining and fully reclining wheelchair.

It must be used with the Postura seat assembly. Check with an Everest and Jennings dealer for feasibility if considering using the Postura legrest cradle with any other type of wheelchair.

The use of the Postura legrest cradle for clients who are able to weight bear when transferring is not recommended because the legrest cradle does not swing away.

To Assemble:

The Postura legrest cradle can be fitted to a 46 cm. (18 in.) adult, 41 cm. (16 in.) narrow adult or Junior 16 wheelchair. It attaches to the Postura adjustable depth seat or the inclinable seat assembly (Refer to Sacral Sitting, Postura Inclinable Seat).

A knob on the side of the legrest cradle adjusts the length from 37 cm. (14.5

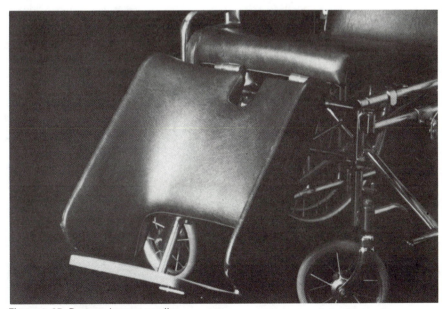

Figure 5-35. Postura legrest cradle.

in.) to 65 cm. (25.5 in.). The legrest cradle is padded and has adjustable elevation.

Above Knee Amputee Cushion

The above knee amputee cushion is a padded wooden seat base plus a padded board that inserts into the seat base. It will provide support and protection for the stump as for example when going through a narrow doorway.

The padded board is removable for occasions when the client is wearing a prothesis or to permit transferring.

The above knee amputee cushion can be constructed for any type of standard adult wheelchair or reclining wheelchair.

Construction:

The above knee amputee cushion is made of 0.6 cm. (0.25 in.) plywood.

1. Cut two seat boards the size of the wheelchair seat. The pieces should be wide enough to sit on the wheelchair seat rails. The corners are rounded.
2. Cut four pieces of 1 cm. (3/8 in.) plywood 1 cm (3/8 in.) wide. Three of the pieces are the same length as the depth of the seat boards minus 2.5 cm. (1 in.). One piece is the same length as the width of the seat boards minus 2.5 cm. (1 in.)
3. The two seat boards and the four plywood strips are assembled according to fig. 5-36. They are secured with glue and screws. Piece 1 is secured in the center of the seat base.
4. The amputee board is made of 0.6 cm. (0.25 in.) plywood. To determine the width of the board: divide the width of the seat base by two and subtract 2 cm. (0.75 in.). To calculate the length of the board, with the client sitting in the wheelchair, measure the length of the stump that is not supported on the seat base, plus the length of the seat base, plus 3 cm. (1.5 in.). The amputee board inserts in space A or B (refer to fig. 5-36) depending on the side of the amputation.
5. The seat base is padded with 5 cm. (2 in.) medium density foam. The section of the amputee board which protrudes from the base is padded

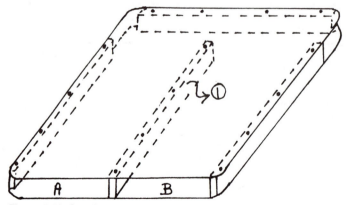

Figure 5-36. Seat base.

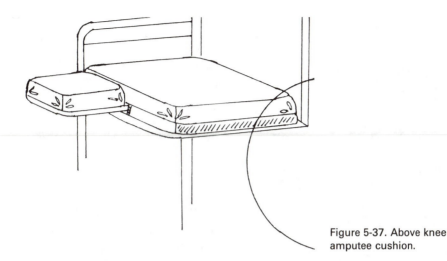

Figure 5-37. Above knee amputee cushion.

with the same foam. The foam is covered with any durable, stretchable fabric. It is stapled to the bottom of the seat base and the amputee board.

Figure "8" Foot Strap

The figure "8" foot strap is used to prevent the foot from falling in front of the footrest due to flaccidity, mild to moderate extensor spasticity or a lack of body awareness.

It is effective in maintaining the foot on the foot plate with the ankle at 90 degrees.

It is not recommended if the foot slips off the foot plate due to plantar flexion deformity.

The figure "8" foot strap can be fitted on any type of footrest or legrest.

Construction:

Use 5 cm. (2 in.) wide webbing, velcro and elastic.

1. Cut the following pieces:
    a. 2 lengths of webbing 22 cm. (8.5 in.) long
    b. 1 length of webbing 45 cm. (18 in.) long

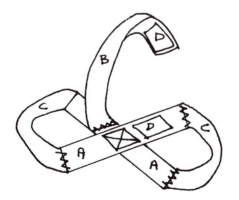

Figure 5-38. Left figure "8" foot strap.

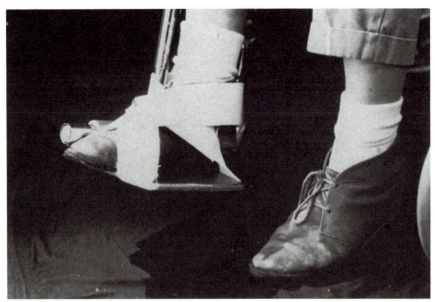

Figure 5-39. Figure "8" foot strap.

      c. 2 lengths of elastic 23 cm. (9 in.) long
      d. 2 lengths of velcro hook and
         loop each 9 cm. (3.5 in.) long
  2. Sew all the pieces together according to Fig. 5-38.

Ankle Positioning Aids

Ankle positioning aids are primarily designed for clients who have plantar flexion contractures of the ankle. They are also used for clients who sit in a reclining wheelchair who need good foot support.

They provide support for the whole foot by adapting to the degree of ankle dorsi flexion required, thus improving sitting stability and the position of the lower extremities.

Construction:

Ankle Positioning Block

Various types of lumber can be used to make the ankle positioning blocks, depending on the height required.

Ankle positioning blocks can be fitted to any type of footrest or elevating legrest.

  1. The length and width of the block is the same as the length and width of the foot plate.
  2. The thin edge of the wedge should be approximately 0.5 cm. (0.25 in.).
  3. To determine the height of the thick edge of the wedge:
     a. For an ankle plantar flexion contracture: With the toes on the foot

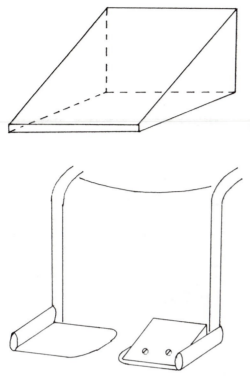

Figure 5-40. Ankle positioning block.

Figure 5-41. Ankle positioning block.

plate and the ankle in as much dorsiflexion as is comfortable, measure the distance from the heel to the foot plate.

   b. To maintain a neutral ankle position: With the heel resting on the foot plate and the ankle at 90 degrees, measure the distance between the toes and the foot plate.

4. The ankle positioning blocks are bolted to the foot plate.

5. The height of the footrest may need to be adjusted.

Foot Plates with Adjustable Angle Setting (Everest and Jennings)

Foot plates with an adjustable angle setting can be fitted to any type of Everest and Jennings legrest or footrest. They may be adapted to other types of wheelchair, depending on the tubing size and method of attachment of the foot plate to the footrest.

The foot plates adjust to dorsiflexion or plantar flexion in varying degrees. The knob on the side of the foot plate adjusts the angle.

Knee Abductor

The knee abductor is used for clients who have increased tone in the adductor muscles of the thigh. It helps prevent adduction contractures and pressure sores on the medial aspect of the knees.

The knee abductor helps to maintain the hips in neutral rotation and keep the pelvis level in order to provide a stable sitting posture.

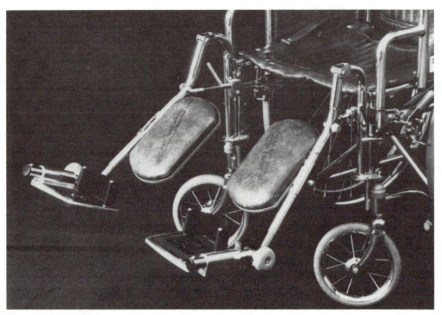

Figure 5-42. Foot plates with adjustable angle setting.

The knee abductor is always positioned between the knees, and not between the thighs, so that adduction is not encouraged by stimulation of the medial aspect of the thighs.

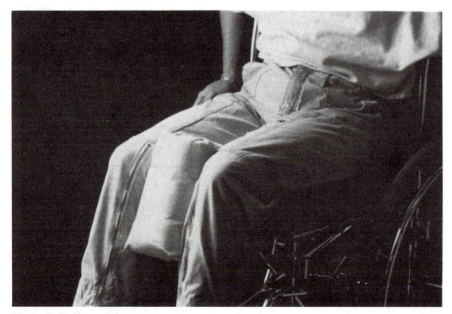

Figure 5-43. Knee abductor.

Construction:

Medium density foam is recommended without the addition of any solid material. This is to minimize the risk of developing a pressure sore on the medial aspect of the knees after prolonged use.

The foam is cut and is rolled into a cylinder 20 cm. (8 in.) long and 15 cm. (6 in.) in diameter, or more, enough to maintain the legs in a neutral position.

A soft and washable fabric is used to cover the knee abductor.

Trunk Support

Good trunk alignment is essential for head and neck control. Eye-hand coordination, eating ability, communication, and participation in day-to-day activities will all be affected.

Poor trunk alignment is likely to cause stress in the back and decrease sitting tolerance.

The trunk must be balanced centrally over the pelvis, the base of support. Stability depends on good muscular support. Physical changes, such as scoliosis, will change the center of gravity and the ability to balance the trunk over the pelvis.

Potential Problems

- Leaning
  When sitting in the wheelchair, the client leans over to one side, forward or backward.
  —This may be caused by slight to severe hypertonicity of certain muscle groups in the trunk which can affect one or both sides.
  —Flaccidity of various muscle groups of the trunk can also cause leaning. One or both sides may be affected to a varying degree and range from minimal to severe involvement.
  —Weakness may also result in leaning.
  —Leaning is often related to fatigue.
  It should be determined whether the client always leans to the same side and how long he/she has been up in the wheelchair when this occurs.
- Pain
  Pain in the back may be caused by poor trunk alignment. It is important to determine when the pain occurs and the cause of the poor trunk alignment.
- Mild to moderate scoliosis which is often accompanied by pain.

Special Considerations

- A wheelchair which is too wide will be unsupportive and promote leaning. The buttocks slide to one side and the client then leans to the other side. One solution is to change the wheelchair for one of an appropriate size (Refer to Part II, Basic Position in a Wheelchair).

- When there is no alternative to using a wheelchair which is too wide, it may be difficult to mobilize the wheelchair using the upper extremities.
- When deciding on the most appropriate trunk support consideration should be given to the client's ability to transfer into the wheelchair and the ability to mobilize the wheelchair.

Possible Solutions

- Side Cushions:
  —Foam side cushions
  —Postura Side Panel (Everest and Jennings)
- Hook-on headrest (Everest and Jennings)
- Semi-reclining or fully reclining wheelchair
- Padded chest restraint:
  —Padded chest restraint
  —Padded chest restraint with shoulder straps
- Posey "Y" wheelchair safety belt (J.T. Posey)
- Otto Bock spherical side thoracic support (Otto Bock)
- Lateral support with padded armrest
- Padded lateral support
- Postura contour back with lateral supports (Everest and Jennings)
- KSS Back with lateral supports (Special Health Systems)
- QA2 Seat Back with thoracic supports (QA2 Seating System)

Side Cushions:

When there is no alternative to using a wheelchair, (which is too wide) the addition of side cushions provide stability by maintaining the pelvis in a centered position.

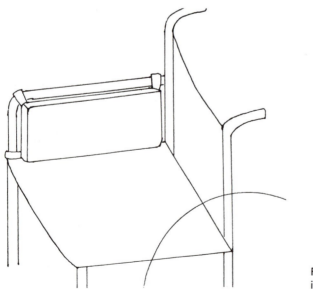

Figure 5-44. Side cushion.

Construction:

Foam Side Cushions

1. To determine the necessary thickness of the side cushions, measure across the widest part of the hips or thighs when the client is seated. Add 2.5 cm. (1 in.).
2. Subtract the width of the wheelchair seat from this measurement.
3. Divide by two to determine the thickness of each side cushion.
4. Measure the length and height inside the armrest to determine the length and width of the cushion.
5. Medium density foam is preferable.
6. Cover the cushions with any type of fabric. Use leatherette when waterproofing is necessary.
7. Sew a length of webbing to the upper corners of each cover to attach the side cushion to the armrest.

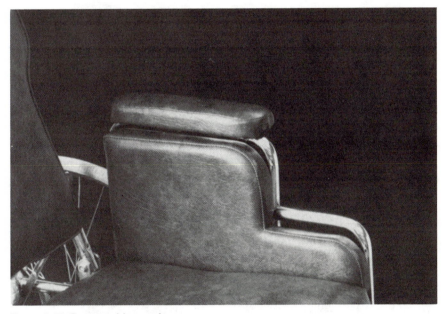

Figure 5-45. Postura side panel.

Postura Side Panel (Everest and Jennings)

Side panels are available from the Postura modular system for full-length or desk-length armrests. They are 2.5 or 5 cm. (1 or 2 in.) thick and are covered with leatherette.

Hook-on Headrest: (Everest and Jennings)

For mild problems of trunk control, the hook-on headrest will provide trunk stability, prevent hyperextension of the upper trunk, head and neck, and provide upper trunk support for tall clients.

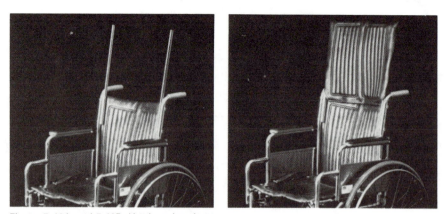

Figure 5-46A and 5-46B. Hook-on headrest.

This type of support does not prevent the client from leaning forward and/or to the side.

The hook-on headrest is used in conjunction with a standard adult wheelchair.

To Assemble:

The metal supports of the hook-on headrest are easily attached to a standard adult wheelchair.

The leatherette cover is available in two standard sizes: 41 cm. (16 in.) wide and 46 cm. (18 in.) wide. It adds 33 cm. (13 in.) to the back height of the wheelchair.

If you wish to make your own cover, use a strong fabric such as leather or leatherette.

Semi-Reclining or Fully Reclining Wheelchair

If the client is using a standard wheelchair and leans forward and/or to the side, and the leaning increases with fatigue, a reclining wheelchair will provide trunk support.

Additional positioning adaptations may be necessary after reassessment of the client.

Padded Chest Restraint

The padded chest restraint is a large foam pad placed over the chest and tied at the back of the wheelchair, preventing forward leaning. It is effective in correcting mild problems of poor trunk posture related to fatigue and/or due to generalized increased tone in the trunk muscles.

This chest restraint does not prevent the client from leaning to the side. If required, padded shoulder straps can be added to the chest restraint to provide extra support to the upper trunk.

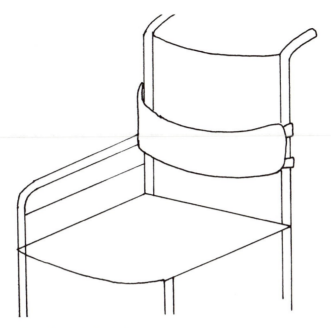

Figure 5-47. Padded chest restraint.

Construction:

Padded Chest Restraint
Use 2.5 cm. (1 in.) low density foam.

1. With the client sitting in the wheelchair, determine the length of foam required by measuring across the chest from one back post to the other. The strip of foam should be about 14 cm. (5.5 in.) wide.
2. The foam is covered with 16 cm. (6.5 in.) wide stockinette or any soft fabric.
3. Four lengths of velcro are sewn, one on each corner, to attach the padded chest restraint to the wheelchair.

Padded Chest Restraint with Shoulder Straps
Use 2.5 cm. (1 in.) low density foam and 5 cm. (2 in.) wide stockinette.

1. Cut two lengths of foam 5 cm. (2 in.) wide and 46 cm. (18 in.) long.
2. Cut two lengths of stockinette 70 cm. (28 in.) long.
3. The two lengths of foam are covered with stockinette.
4. The shoulder straps are sewn on the top and in the middle of the padded chest restraint 6 cm. (2.5 in.) apart.
5. Velcro is sewn on the other end of the shoulder strap to attach it to the wheelchair's rear handles.
6. The shoulder straps cross at the back behind the neck.

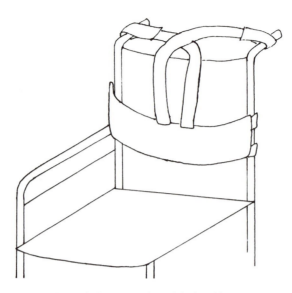

Figure 5-48. Padded chest restraint with shoulder straps.

Posey "Y" Wheelchair Safety Belt (J.T. Posey)

The Posey "Y" wheelchair safety belt is used as a reminder to discourage leaning forward. This safety belt is effective with clients who lean forward but who are able to correct their position.

It is ineffective when the leaning is caused by fatigue and trunk weakness and will not prevent side leaning.

It comes in one adult size but is easily adjustable to most sizes and fits most types of wheelchair. The "Y" belt is made of strong washable webbing.

To Assemble:

The two top straps of the "Y" belt go over the shoulders and attach to the rear handles. A second long belt runs through a hole in the bottom of the "Y" belt and crosses at the back of the wheelchair attaching to the kick spurs. It is easy to put on or remove.

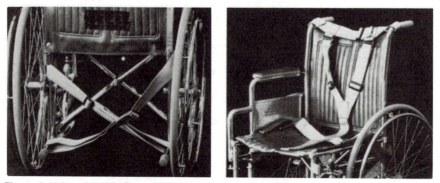

Figure 5-49A and 5-49B. Posey "Y" wheelchair safety belt.

Otto Bock Spherical Side Thoracic Support (Otto Bock)

This thoracic support prevents leaning to one side, especially when leaning is due to hypertonicity of the trunk muscles. This support may slow the progression of a scoliosis or correct a mild one.

It is not recommended when leaning is fatigue-related and due to weakness of the trunk muscles for the client who uses a standard wheelchair. It will not prevent the client from leaning forward.

The use of this support will not affect the method of transfer because the support pad can be raised and swung to the side. When supporting the client it locks in place. Movement of the upper extremities is not impeded by the support.

To Assemble:

The spherical thoracic supports can be fitted to the back post or armrest of any type of wheelchair. They are fully and easily adjustable to accommodate any body build.

The support pads are available in three sizes: small, medium, and large. The three styles of rod assembly— regular, extended, and dropped—are adapted specifically for right or left sides. Various sizes of mounting hardware are available to accommodate different sizes of back posts. The thoracic supports can be used singly or as a pair depending on the client's needs.

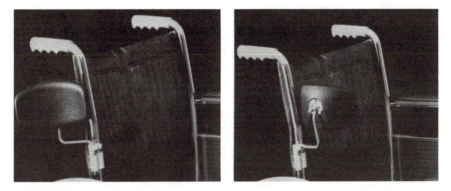

Figure 5-50A and 5-50B. Otto Bock spherical side thoracic support with large size support pad and right regular rod assembly.

Lateral Support With Padded Armrest:

This lateral support is used when leaning to the side is due to hypertonicity of muscles of the trunk. It is also effective in preventing mild to moderate slumping to the side due to weakness of trunk muscles. The leaning may be related to fatigue.

It provides good support to the upper extremity but does not permit functional use of the arm. It does not prevent leaning forward.

The lateral support with padded armrest can be fitted on a standard adult wheelchair, or a semi-reclining or fully-reclining wheelchair.

Construction:

Use 1 cm. (3/8 in.) plywood.

1. Cut the following pieces:

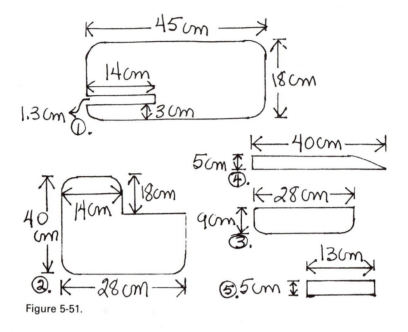

Figure 5-51.

2. Piece 2 fits in the slot in piece 1. They are fixed together with two 3 cm. (1.25 in.) corner braces and screws.
3. Pieces 4 and 5 are fixed to piece 1 with screws and glue.
4. Piece 3 is fixed to piece 1 with two corner braces and screws. Piece 3 is 5.5 cm. (2.25 in.) from piece 2.

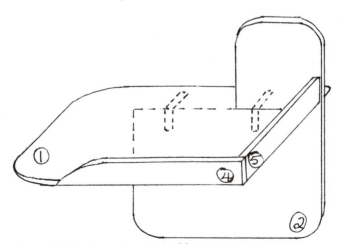

Figure 5-52. Left lateral support with armrest.

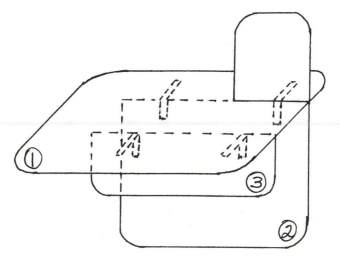

Figure 5-53. Left lateral support with armrest.

5. The lateral support with armrest is padded with 2.5 cm. (1 in.) low density foam. The foam is stapled to the lateral support with armrest.
6. The lateral support with padded armrest can be covered with any durable fabric such as denim. The cover is stapled to the lateral support with armrest.

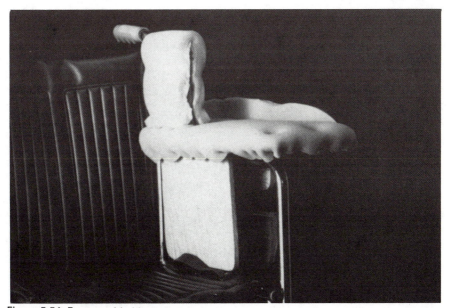

Figure 5-54. Foam padded lateral suport with armrest.

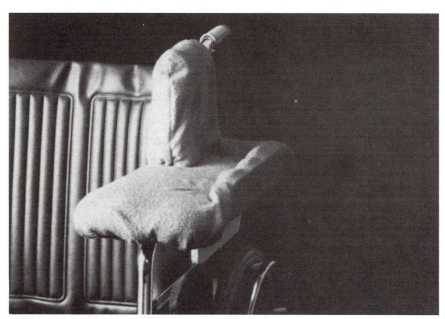

Figure 5-55. Lateral support with padded armrest.

Padded Lateral Support:

If the client leans to the side from fatigue, the padded lateral support is recommended. This type of support is not intended for clients who are able to mobilize the wheelchair with their upper extremities, although the use of the upper extremities for table activities will not be limited. Vision to the side may be restricted.

The lateral support may be used singly or as a pair and can be fitted to most types of adult wheelchair.

Construction:

Use 1 cm. (3/8 in.) plywood.

1. Cut the following pieces:

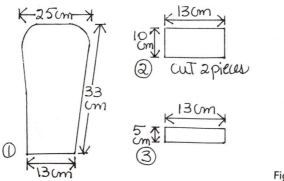

Figure 5-56.

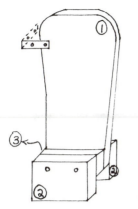

Figure 5-57. Right lateral support.

2. Piece 1 has a slight angle to accommodate the angle on the back post of the standard adult wheelchair. To determine the angle, draw a line on cardboard along the back post from the rear handle to the armrest (the pad is removed) with the base of the cardboard resting on the armrest. The reclining wheelchair does not have any angle to the back post.
3. Pieces 1, 2 and 3 are fixed together with two 5 cm. (2 in.) long bolts. The nuts are on the outside of the support.
4. A 3 cm. (1.25 in.) corner brace is bolted so it lines up with a screw situated on the back post leaving a space the thickness of the post (Refer to Fig. 5-57).
5. The lateral support is padded with 2.5 cm. (1 in.) low density foam. Cover with any durable fabric such as denim. The cover is stapled to the lateral support.

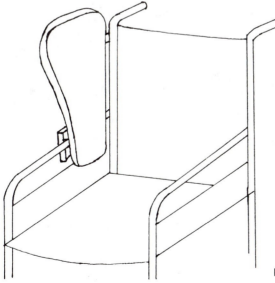

Figure 5-58. Right lateral support.

6. The padded lateral support sits on the armrest and is fixed to the back post using the screw from the back upholstery and the corner brace.
7. Pieces 2 (Refer to Fig. 5-56) should be longer if the lateral support is fitted to a reclining wheelchair.

Postura Contour Back With Lateral Supports (Everest and Jennings)

The Postura contour back with lateral supports is recommended for controlling mild positioning problems of leaning to the side due to poor trunk control. It is more effective if used on a reclining wheelchair.

The lateral support does not limit the use of the upper extremities and can be used singly or as a pair. They are independently and easily adjustable in height, width, and rotation.

The Postura back with lateral supports can be fitted to most Everest and Jennings reclining wheelchairs and standard wheelchairs with detachable armrests. The Postura contour back may be compatible with other types of wheelchair, but it is advisable to consult a local dealer for feasibility.

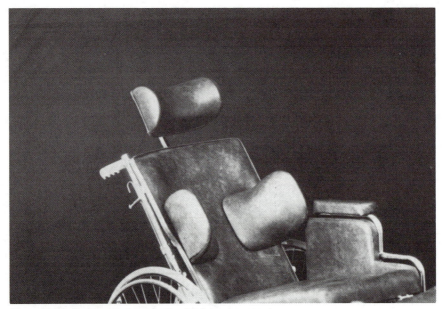

Figure 5-59. Postura contour back with lateral supports.

KSS Back With Lateral Supports (Special Health Systems):

The KSS back with lateral supports is effective in controlling moderate positioning problems of leaning to the side due to poor trunk control. It may slow the progression of a scoliosis or correct a mild one. Firm support is provided to the upper body while allowing unrestricted use of the upper extremities.

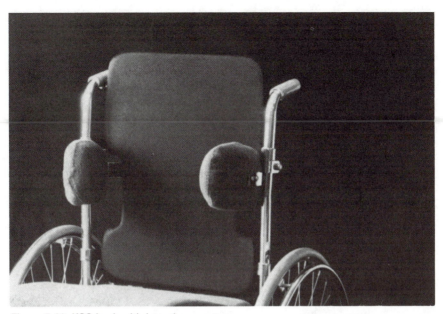

Figure 5-60. KSS back with lateral supports.

The lateral support attaches to the KSS back with a steel bracket and can be used individually or as a pair. They are adjustable in width by 1.23 cm. (0.5 in.) increments. Height adjustment is done by elevating or lowering the KSS back (Refer to Back Support KSS Back)

The lateral support is padded with a 2.5 cm. (1 in.) medium density foam or a 2.5 cm. (1 in.) contouring foam. It is covered with lycra and has a removable stretch terry cover.

QA2 Seat Back With Thoracic Supports (QA2 Seating System)

The QA2 seat back with thoracic supports can be used with clients who are at risk for side leaning or who are leaning slightly to the side due to poor trunk control.

Minimal support is provided by this system and it is often more effective if used in conjunction with a reclining wheelchair.

The QA2 seat back with thoracic support can be fitted to most types of standard adult wheelchair and reclining wheelchair with widths ranging from 36 cm. (14 in.) to 51 cm. (20 in.).

To Assemble:

The QA2 seat back is used with the regular or drop seat base (refer to Buttocks, QA2 Seat Base, QA2 Drop Seat Base). The QA2 seating system is made of strong ABS thermal plastic.

Trunk support is provided and custom fitting is possible as the two thoracic supports are attached to the seat back with dual-lock (a type of industrial velcro).

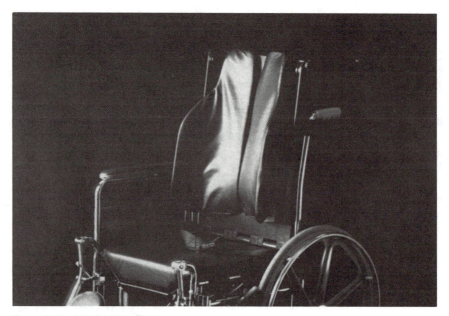

Figure 5-61. QA2 Seating System.

With the sling seat removed the seating system inserts into the wheelchair. A strap secures the seat back to the wheelchair.

Back Support

Good back support prevents and/or minimizes back pain and improves comfort, especially for clients with conditions such as scoliosis or osteoporosis where the integrity of the spine is destroyed. Sitting tolerance increases as pain decreases, and improvement in feelings of well-being are likely. The need for pain medication may be decreased or alleviated.

The back supports described are not intended to correct spinal deformities, but rather to accommodate them in order to improve comfort and sitting tolerance.

Potential Problems

- Back Pain
- Poor Sitting Tolerance

    Scoliosis, kyphosis or decreased lumbar curvature affect the integrity and alignment of the spinal vertebrae, causing back pain and poor sitting tolerance.

    Bending of the trunk is thought to be a contributing factor of compression fractures on the spinal vertebrae.

    Back pain and poor sitting tolerance may also be due to osteoarthritis or osteoporosis with or without compression fractures of vertebrae.

    When assessing the client, note any position that provides relief from the pain; the part of the back in which the pain occurs; and the sitting tolerance.

- Pressure Sores
  Pressure sores may occur over prominent spinal processes.

Special Considerations

- The addition of a back cushion to a wheelchair decreases the depth of the seat.
  According to the thickness of the cushion provided, the client may feel insecure as body weight is moved forward and less support is given to the thighs.
  A custom made wheelchair with a longer seat depth may be indicated.
- Increasing the height of the seat back may impede mobilization of the wheelchair with the upper extremities.

Possible Solutions

- Back Cushion
- Fully-reclining of semi-reclining wheelchairs
- Lumbar backrest cushion
  —Lumbar backrest foam cushion
  —Jay Combi contoured backrest (Jay Medical Ltd.)
- Soft T-Foam back cushion
- Firm contour back supports
  —Postura contour back (Everest and Jennings)
  —QA2 Seating System (QA2 Seating System)
  —KSS Back (Special Health Systems)

Back Cushion

The purpose of a back cushion is to improve comfort. Sitting tolerance may increase as back pain is controlled.

A back cushion may be an effective solution for clients who complain of back pain but do not suffer from spinal deformities which would require additional support.

There is no special way to determine which type of cushion is the most appropriate. Personal preference for a soft or firm cushion may be indicated by the client. The most appropriate type of cushion will be determined by trial and error.

Back cushions can be fitted to any type of wheelchair and should be secured usually to the back frame to prevent slipping.

Construction:

Use 2.5 cm. (1 in.) low or medium density foam depending on how firm a cushion is required. Egg crate foam 2.5 cm. (1 in.) low density can be used for a soft back cushion.

1. The cushion is cut to the size of the wheelchair's back upholstery.
2. A soft and stretchy fabric is used to cover the foam cushion.

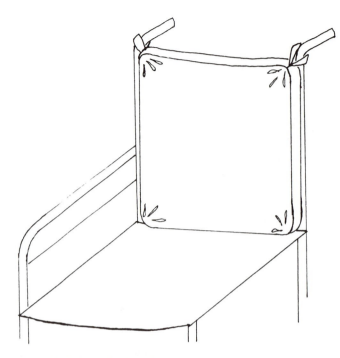

Figure 5-62. Foam back cushion.

3. Two lengths of webbing are sewn to the upper corners to attach the back cushion to the rear handles of the wheelchair.

Fully-Reclining or Semi-Reclining Wheelchairs

To eliminate some of the effects of gravity on the spine, a reclining wheelchair may be used to alleviate back pain or to improve trunk alignment.

It is important to maintain the angle of hip and trunk at 100 degrees in a reclining wheelchair to prevent sliding forward and skin breakdown from the shearing force. A wedge cushion is effective for this purpose.

Lumbar Backrest Cushion

This cushion provides support to the lumbar region. It assists in restoring the natural lumbar curve thus promoting improved posture. It helps to reduce fatigue and decrease back pain.

The lumbar cushion can be fitted on any type of wheelchair.

Construction:

Lumbar Backrest Foam Cushion

Use 2.5 cm. or 5 cm. (1 or 2 in.) low density foam, depending on the client need. Eggcrate foam can also be used.

1. It is usually 20 cm (8 in.) high and is cut to fit the width of the wheelchair.
2. It is covered with stockinette or any soft and stretchy fabric.

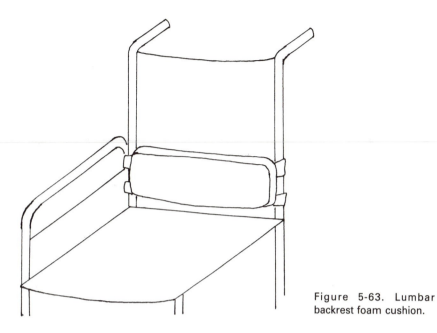

Figure 5-63. Lumbar backrest foam cushion.

3. Four lengths of velcro are sewn one in each corner to attach the cushion to the wheelchair.

Jay Combi Contoured Backrest (Jay Medical, Ltd.)

The Combi contoured backrest is made of low density foam and has a removable foam insert for custom fitting.

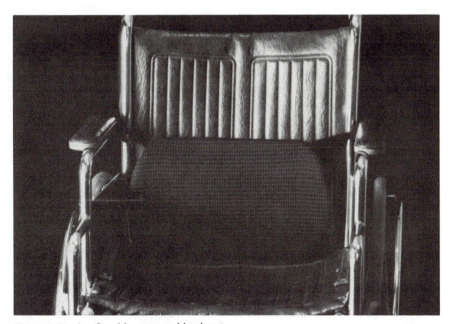

Figure 5-64. Jay Combi contoured backrest.

Soft T-Foam Back Cushion

This back cushion is made of soft T-foam which molds to accommodate bony prominences of the spine. It helps prevent pressure sores and improves sitting comfort.

Construction:

Use 1.3 or 2.5 cm. (0.5 or 1 in.) soft T-foam. It is usually cut to fit the size of the back of the wheelchair.

The cushion can be covered with any soft and stretchy fabric. It is attached to the wheelchair with ties which are sewn in the upper corners of the cover.

Firm Contour Back Supports

The hammock backrest of the wheelchair promotes lumbar kyphosis which is a rounding-out of the lower spine. With this condition the tendency to slide down, forward and out of the wheelchair is increased. The hammock effect of the backrest may contribute to increased back pain and poor sitting tolerance of clients with conditions such as osteoporosis, osteoarthritis and compression fractures of the vertebrae.

A rigid back support assists in promoting good alignment of the spine and in providing firm support to the trunk. Thus back pain is decreased and sitting tolerance improved.

A firm back support should not be given to a client without also providing a firm seat base in order to maintain a level pelvis.

To Assemble:

Postura Contour Back (Everest and Jennings)

The Postura contour back can be fitted to most Everest and Jennings standard adult wheelchairs with detachable armrests, semi-reclining or fully reclining wheelchairs. It is available in two adult sizes: adult 46 cm. (18 in.) and narrow adult 41 cm. (16 in.). When considering using the Postura contour back with a type of wheelchair other than Everest and Jennings consult a local dealer for feasibility.

QA2 Seating System (QA2 Seating System)

This system includes a regular or drop seat base and seat back.

The two thoracic supports are adjustable for added trunk support and good custom fitting.

To assemble refer to Trunk Support, QA2 Seat back with thoracic supports.

KSS Back (Special Health Systems)

The KSS Back can be fitted on most standard adult wheelchairs and semi-reclining or fully-reclining wheelchairs. It is available in two standard adult sizes: 46 cm. (18 in.) and 41 cm. (16 in.) wide.

The KSS Back suspends with slight reclination on the vertical bars of the

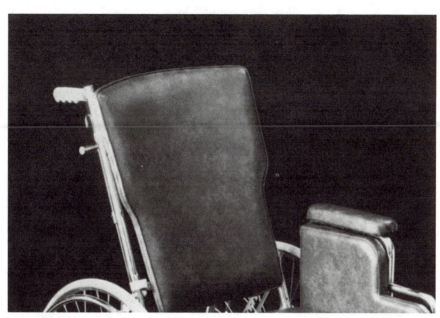

Figure 5-65. Postura contour back.

wheelchair. It is held in place by two "anti-gravity hooks" that permit adjustment for proper height.

The back is padded with a 2.5 cm. (1 in.) medium density foam and has a lycra cover.

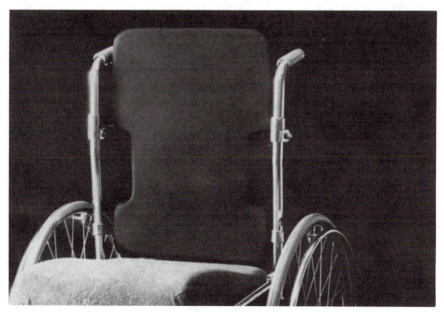

Figure 5-66. KSS back.

Head and Neck

Positioning of the head and neck relies on good body position and in particular trunk stability.

The ability to maintain good head and neck position affects the performance of activities such as the time spent eating, behavior during eating, independent eating, and the ability to keep food and liquid in the mouth. Position of the head also affects swallowing and the risk of choking.

Communication with friends and family is difficult without the ability to maintain an upright position of the head in order to make eye contact.

Eye-hand coordination needed for recreational activities, such as table games, also requires head control.

Potential Problems

- Poor Head Control
  The head may droop forward, to one side, and/or fall back into an hyper-extended position.
  A drooping head may result from weakness and/or fatigue. It may also be caused by a slight to severe decrease or increase in the tone of the muscles of the neck and could affect one side more than the other. Paralysis of the extensor muscles of the neck also causes a drooping head.
  It should be noted whether the head always droops in the same direction and when it occurs.
- Pain
  The client may complain of pain in the neck and upper back. It may be related to poor head righting or a condition such as arthritis of the vertebrae. The assessment should note whether the pain occurs with movement, is accentuated by fatigue and/or whether it is constantly present.

Special Considerations

- A rigid cervical collar is usually effective in maintaining proper alignment of the head, but it may be uncomfortable and interfere with speaking and swallowing.
- A supportive headband attached to the wheelchair may not be acceptable to client or family for aesthetic reasons.

Possible Solutions.

- Foam headrest
- Back extension on standard adult wheelchair (Everest and Jennings)
- Semi-reclining or fully-reclining wheelchair
- Pillow headrest
- Crown head support
  —Wooden crown head support
  —Crown head support with Otto Bock headrest attachment (Otto Bock)

- Head and neck supports—Seating Systems:
  —Postura Headrest supports (Everest and Jennings)
  —QA2 Headrest (QA2 Seating System)
  —KSS neck support (Special Health Systems)
  —Otto Bock head and neck supports (Otto Bock)

Foam Headrest

When poor head control and limited strength cause the head to fall into an hyperextended position, and/or fall to the side, the foam headrest can provide support for mild to moderate positioning problems.

This type of headrest is used in conjunction with a fully reclining or semi-reclining wheelchair with a detachable telescopic headrest.

If the head continues to droop forward when the client is positioned, in a reclining wheelchair, the foam headrest will be ineffective.

Construction:

Use 2 layers of 7.5 cm. (3 in.) medium density foam.

1. Two pieces of foam 24 cm. (9 in.) high by 37 cm. (14 in.) wide are glued together to form a block.
2. The block is carved to provide contour fitting for the head and neck following the measurements in the diagram. The headrest is 9 cm. (3.5 in.) thick in the middle at the bottom.
3. The measurements can be modified to fit the individual client.
4. The headrest can be covered with 17 cm. (6.5 in.) wide stockinette or any soft and stretchy fabric.

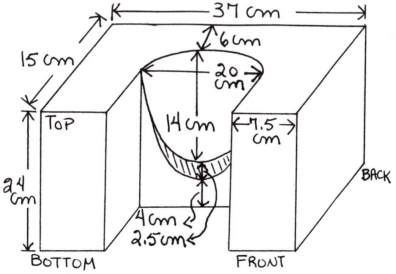

Figure 5-67. Foam headrest.

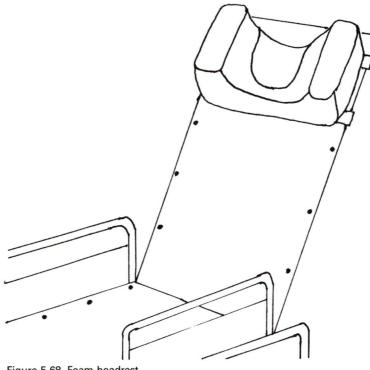

Figure 5-68. Foam headrest.

An elastic is sewn to the two sides of the cover to secure the headrest to the wheelchair.

Back Extension on Standard Adult Wheelchair (Everest and Jennings)

The back extension is an effective support when used for problems of mild to moderate hypertonicity of the extensor muscles of the neck which causes the head to fall back.

It is also used to prevent poor head righting due to fatigue by providing support for the head, neck and upper trunk.

To Assemble:
Refer to Trunk support, Hook-on-Headrest.

Semi-Reclining or Fully-Reclining Wheelchair

A reclining wheelchair with a detachable telescopic headrest can be an effective solution for the client whose head falls forward or to the side, due to decreased tone in the extensor muscles of the neck or weakness of the muscles of the neck. The inability to maintain the head in an upright position may increase with fatigue.

The effect of gravity will hold the head back on the headrest, which should be provided together with the reclining wheelchair.

Additional support such as a foam headrest may be needed to complete the positioning.

Pillow Headrest

A pillow headrest is recommended when minimal support will provide comfort.

A pillow headrest secured to the detachable telescopic headrest of a reclining wheelchair will help to hold the head in an upright position.

Construction:

1. The open end of the pillow case is held together with velcro so the pillow case can be easily removed and washed.
2. Two lengths of elastic 2.5 cm. (1 in.) wide are sewn onto the ends of the pillow case to hold the pillow on the headrest. One length of elastic joins the upper corners and one joins the lower corners.

Crown Head Support

Clients who are unable to keep the head from drooping forward may find the crown head support useful and may learn to put it on independently when they need the extra support.

It is usually used in conjunction with a standard adult wheelchair.

Construction:

Wooden Crown Head Support

For a 46 cm. (18 in.) wide adult wheelchair.
Base: Use 1 cm. (3/8 in.) plywood for the base.

1. In the center at the top of a 20 cm. x 48 cm. (7.75 in. x 19 in.) board, attach a box 13 cm. x 5 cm. x 5 cm. (5 in. x 2 in. x 2 in.) (Refer to Fig 5-68)

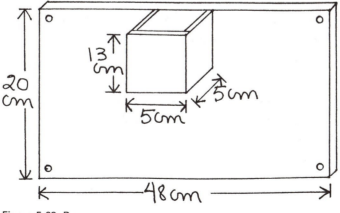

Figure 5-69. Base.

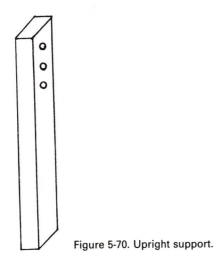

Figure 5-70. Upright support.

2. One hole is made in each corner of the board. to attach it to the back of the wheelchair. These screw holes must line up with the screws on the back of the wheelchair.

Upright support:

On a wooden post 56 cm. x 2.5 cm. x 4 cm. (22 in. x 1 in. x 1.5 in.), drill 3 holes large enough for a 5 cm. (2 in.) long bolt. They start 2.5 cm. (1 in.) form the top and are 4 cm. (1.5 in.) apart.

Head Band:

The head band is in two parts: attachment and crown.

Attachment:

Use two pieces of a low temperature thermo-plastic material, such as san-splint 25 x 6.5 cm (10 x 2.5 in.) in size. Make three holes in each piece of san-splint 2.5 cm. (1 in.) apart at one end and one hole at 2.5 cm. (1 in.) from the other end.

Crown:

Use one piece of 1.2 cm. (0.5 in.) low-temperature, closed-cell foam material, such as plastazote, cut 76 x 7.5 cm (30 x 3 in.) in size. Make one hole 4 cm. (1.5 in.) from each end. The holes on the plastazote need to be reinforced with a piece 5 x 5 cm. (2 x 2 in.) of any type of thin plastic. The platazote can be covered with stockinette and changed as necessary for cleanliness.

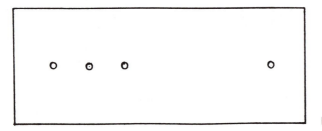

Figure 5-71. Attachment.

To assemble the head support:

1. The board is fixed on the wheelchair
2. The post is put in the box
3. The two pieces of san-splint are fixed to the post with a 10 cm. (4 in.) long bolt. The 3 holes on the post and the san-splint are for adjustments.
4. The plastazote head band is fixed to the san-splint with a 5 cm. (2 in.) long bolt. A 20 cm. (8 in.) long piece of webbing can be sewn on the stockinette to keep the head band from falling down over the face.

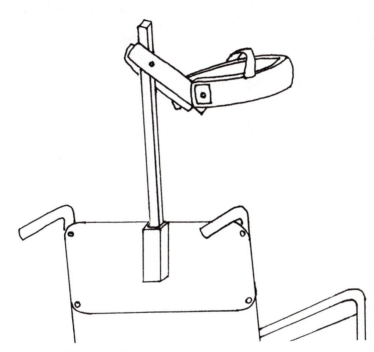

Figure 5-72. Wooden Crown head support.

Crown Head Support with Otto Bock Headrest Attachment (Otto Bock)

An alternative to the wooden crown head support is to use the wheelchair adapter kit with the headrest—multi- or single-axis straight or offset—from Otto Bock (Refer to Fig. 5-73).

The wheelchair adapter kit can be fitted on any type of adult wheelchair with widths ranging from 36 cm. to 46 cm. (14 to 18 in.).

The headrest hardware can be multi- or single-axis, straight or offset, depending on the amount of adjustment needed. The single-axis straight or offset hardware is adjustable in height and depth. The hardware multi-axis straight or offset provides a full range of adjustment in all three planes.

The plastazote head band described above can be easily fitted to the axis with a piece of san-splint 5 cm. x 41 cm. (2 x 16 in.) molded to fit the axis.

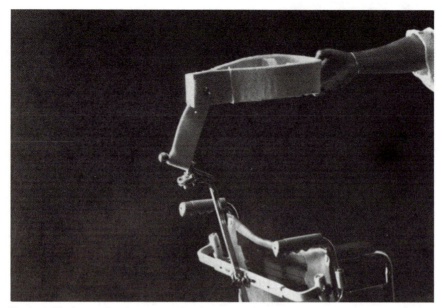

Figure 5-73. Crown Head support with Otto Bock multi-axis offset headrest attachment.

A bolt 5 cm. (2 in.) long is used to fix the head band to the piece of san-splint.

Head and Neck Supports—Seating Systems:

There are four types of fully adjustable head and neckrest supports which are part of a complete seating systems:

- Postura Headrest supports
- QA2 Headrest
- KSS Neck support
- Otto Bock Head and Neck supports

They are recommended for any type of positioning problem of the head or neck except for that of the head which droops forward.

To Assemble:

Postura Headrest Supports (Everest and Jennings)

The Postura Headrests are adjustable in height, depth, and angle.

There are three styles of headrest available: concave headrest, deep concave headrest, and neckrest.

The concave headrest provides full head support. The deep concave headrest is used for additional lateral support. The neckrest is designed to provide support to the cervical vertebrae. The Postura headrest support is used in conjunction with the Postura contour back. For the fitting of the contour back, refer to Back Support, Postura Contour Back.

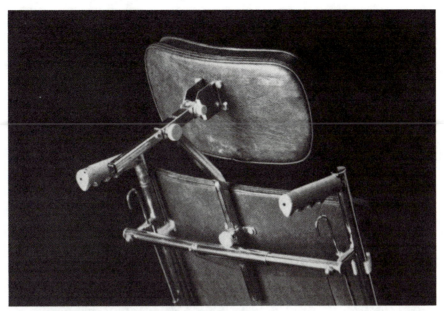

Figure 5-74. Postura contour back with headrest.

QA2 Headrest (QA2 Seating System)

The QA2 headrest is fully adjustable in height, depth, and angle. The headrest hardware assembly can be fitted with any type of Otto Bock headrest cushion.

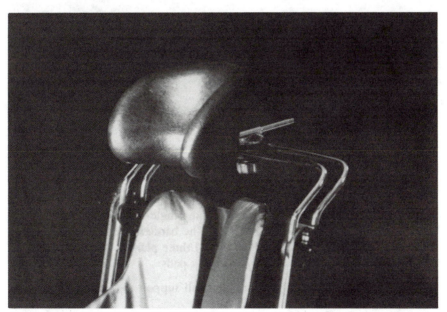

Figure 5-75. QA2 Headrest with combination head and neckrest Otto Bock cushion.

The headrest is used in conjunction with the QA2 Seat and Back. For the fitting of the seat and back, refer to Trunk Support, QA2 Seat Back with thoracic supports.

KSS Neck Support (Special Health Systems)

The KSS neck support is easily adjustable in height and depth. Designed to provide support to the neck and lower head, it prevents hyperextension and permits lateral movement of the head.

The contoured plastic neck pad has 2.5 cm. (1 in.) medium density foam padding. It is covered with lycra and has a removable stretch terry cloth cover.

The KSS neck support is used in conjunction with the KSS Back. For the fitting of the back refer to Back Support, KSS Back.

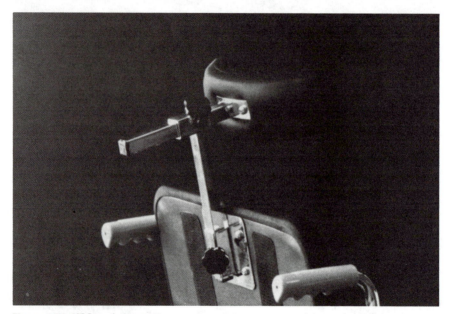

Figure 5-76. KSS neck support.

Otto Bock Head and Neck Supports (Otto Bock)

The Otto Bock head and neck supports can be fitted on any adult wheelchair of width ranging from 36 cm. to 46 cm. (14 to 18 in.) wide using the wheelchair adapter kit.

The headrest hardware can be multi- or single-axis, straight, or offset, depending on the amount of adjustment needed. The single-axis straight or offset is hardware adjustable in height and depth. The hardware multi-axis straight or offset provide full range of adjustment in all three planes.

Otto Bock offers a wide variety of support pads:

—combination head/neckrest: provides full support to the head and neck.
    It also gives lateral support.

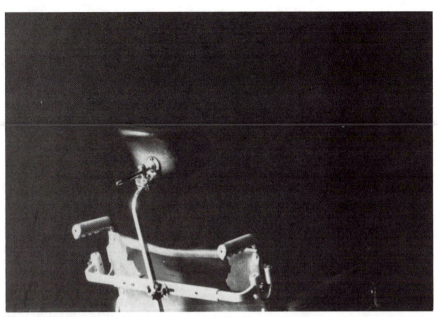

Figure 5-77. Otto Bock wheelchair adapter kit with multi-axis offset headrest hardware and combination head/neckrest support pad.

—Neckrest (small, large or tapered): provides support to the neck and the lower head.
—Headrest (small and large): provides support to the head only and does not restrict lateral movement.

Upper Extremities

The position of the upper extremities affects hand function. To maximize independence in activities of daily living, such as self-care, meal management and mobilization of the wheelchair, the upper extremity must have adequate support.

Intervention is necessary to position the nonfunctional upper extremity for the protection of joint integrity, control muscle tone, prevention of contractures, and/or alleviation of pain.

Potential Problems

One or more of the following problems may exist simultaneously:

- Subluxation of the shoulder joint:
  Subluxation refers to the presence of a space between the acromion process and the head of the humerus. The integrity of the joint is dependent upon muscular support. If the muscles are weak, ligaments stretch and the joint capsule is weakened, resulting in subluxation of the joint. Shoulder subluxation is often accompanied by pain.

- Flaccidity which may be slight to severe.
- Spasticity which may be slight to severe.
- Weakness of individual muscle groups or of the whole extremity.
- Oedema which usually occurs in the hand and may extend up the wrist.
- Contractures: Flexion contractures are common and may involve one or more joints.
- Perceptual deficit such as decreased awareness of an arm and/or visual deficit such as hemianopsia which result in the inability to see one side of the body.
  Fingers may get caught in the spokes of the wheel or an arm may be crushed between the wheelchair and a wall or doorway.
- Impaired sensitivity in the affected upper extremity.

Special Considerations

- The method used to transfer the client must be considered when using a wheelchair table as an aid to positioning the upper extremity, as it will impede independent transferring.
- Mobility may be restricted when using a wheelchair table. Using the unaffected extremity to reach and push the hand rim will be difficult when the wheelchair table extends past the armrests.
- The use of a wheelchair table which does not permit the client to see the lower extremities may increase perceptual problems and enhance lack of body awareness.
- It is often difficult for a client to get close to the table when using an arm trough due to its size and position on the wheelchair. The adaptation may not be acceptable for this reason. It is important to discuss with the client the necessity of the arm trough or other proposed adaptations.
- Functional use of the affected upper extremity must be carefully assessed when deciding on the most appropriate type of support.

Possible Solutions

- Padded armrest
- Flat padded armrest
- Molded armrest
- Elevating molded armrest
- Otto bock armrests (Otto Bock)
- Wheelchair table:
  —Wooden wheelchair table
  —Clear lap tray (Special Health Systems)

Padded Armrest

The padded armrest is designed to provide good support to the affected upper extremity, especially to the shoulder.

It is usually ineffective when there is severe spasticity of the upper extremity as the arm tends to be held close to the chest and consequently off the armrest.

It may be inappropriate for clients who have severe heminegligence, as the limb will not be positioned within the visual field.

This type of armrest can be easily fitted to any type of adult wheelchair which has full length armrests, and it is easily removed.

Construction:

The padded armrest is made of 1 cm. (3/8 in.) plywood.

1. Cut the following pieces:

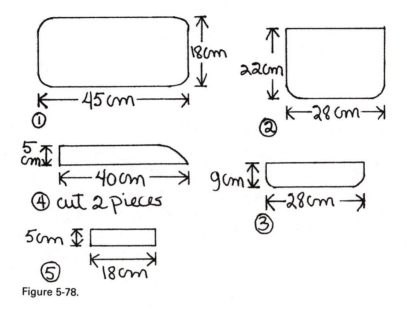

Figure 5-78.

2. Piece 2 is 3 cm. (1.25 in.) from the edge of piece 1. Piece 2 is fixed to piece 1 with two 3 cm. (1.25 in.) corner braces and screws.
   Piece 3 is 5.5 cm. (2.25 in.) from piece 2. Piece 3 is fixed to piece 1 with two 3 cm (1.25 in.) corner braces and screws.
3. Pieces 4 and 5 are fixed to piece 1 with glue and screws.

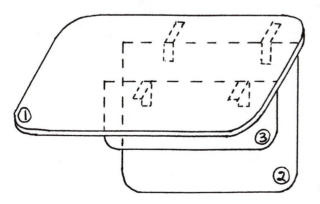

Figure 5-79. Left armrest.

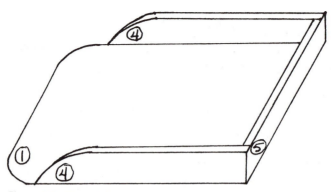

Figure 5-80. Top of the armrest.

4. The armrest is padded with 2.5 cm. (1 in.) low-density foam. The foam is stapled to the armrest.
5. The padded armrest can be covered with any resistant fabric, such as denim. The cover is stapled to the armrest.

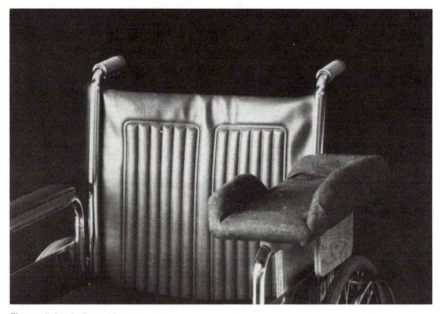

Figure 5-81. Left padded armrest.

Flat Padded Armrest

The flat padded armrest provides good support for the weak or flaccid upper extremity and especially to the shoulder. It is also recommended in cases of mild spasticity of the upper limb.

On this support the arm is held within the immediate visual field. It can be easily fitted to any type of wheelchair with full length armrests and can be easily removed.

Construction:

The flat padded armrest is made of 1 cm. (3/8 in.) plywood.

1. Cut the following pieces:

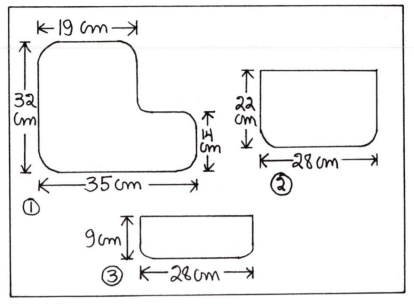

Figure 5-82.

2. Piece 2 is 3 cm. (1.25 in.) from the edge of piece 1. Piece 2 is fixed to piece 1 with two 3 cm (1.25 in.) corner braces and screws.
   Piece 3 is 5.5 cm. (2.25 in.) from piece 2. Piece 2 is fixed to piece 1 with two 3 cm. (1.25 in.) corner braces and screws.
3. The flat armrest is padded with 2.5 cm. (1 in.) low-density foam.

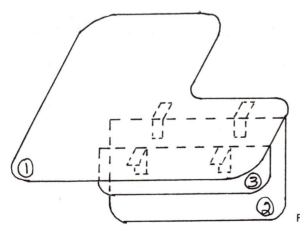

Figure 5-83. Left flat armrest.

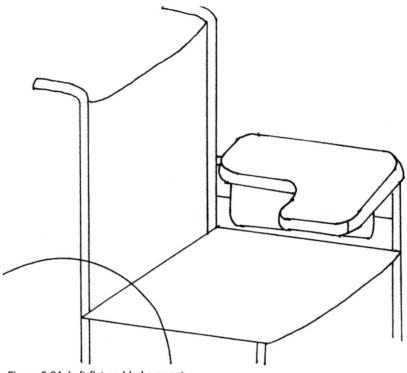

Figure 5-84. Left flat padded armrest.

4. The flat padded armrest can be covered with any resistant fabric, such as denim. The cover is stapled to the armrest.

Molded Armrest

The molded armrest provides good support to the affected upper extremity, especially to the shoulder.

It is usually ineffective when there is severe spasticity of the upper extremity because the arm tends to be held close to the chest and consequently off the armrest.

It may be inappropriate for clients with severe heminegligence as the affected extremity will not be held within the visual field.

The molded armrest can be fitted to any type of adult wheelchair which has full length armrests.

Although the molded armrest is easily removed from the wheelchair it is usually left in place because it does not restrict transfers.

Construction:

The molded armrest is made of a strong, thick, high-temperature thermoplastic material such as Uvex 0.3 cm. (1/8 in.)

1. Cut the following piece:

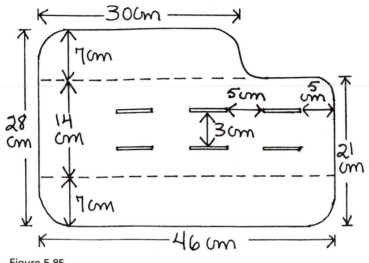

Figure 5-85.

Six slots 5.5 cm. × 0.5 cm. (2.25 in. × 1/5 in.) are cut.

2. Using a 14 cm. × 7 cm. × 46 cm. (5.5 in. × 2.75 in. × 18 in.) wooden block, mold the armrest to bend the two outer sides at 90 degree angles.

3. Make three straps with 5 cm. (2 in.) wide webbing, velcro and 5 cm. (2 in.) long stainless "D" rings. The length of webbing used is 27 cm. (10.5 in.). The overall length of the finished strap is 23 cm. (9 in.)

   The three webbing straps fit in the slots of the armrest to fix the armrest to the wheelchair.

4. A foam pad of 14 cm. × 46 cm. (5.5 in. × 18 in.) is made of 2.5 cm. (1 in.) low-density foam. The foam pad is covered with a thin, stretchable fabric such as stockinette.

   The foam pad is added to the armrest for comfort.

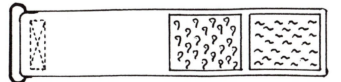

Figure 5-86. Webbing strap.

Elevating Molded Armrest

The elevating armrest is designed to control oedema in the hand.

It can be fitted to any type of adult wheelchair which has full length armrests.

Although the elevating armrest is easily removed, it is usually left in place because it does not restrict transfers.

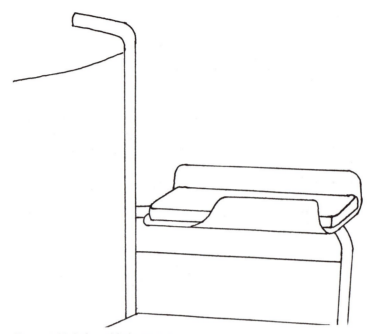

Figure 5-87. Left molded armrest.

Construction:

The elevating armrest is constructed in the same way as the molded armrest, with an added small wooden bridge to provide the elevation.

The wooden bridge is made of 2.5 cm. (1 in.) thick wood.

1. Cut the following piece:

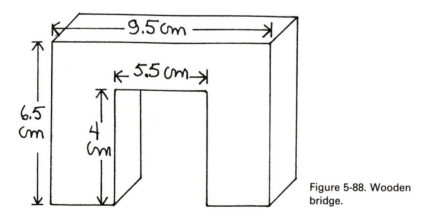

Figure 5-88. Wooden bridge.

2. The bridge is fixed to the molded armrest with two screws and rests on the armrest pad of the wheelchair.

The closer the bridge is placed to the elbow, the greater will be the

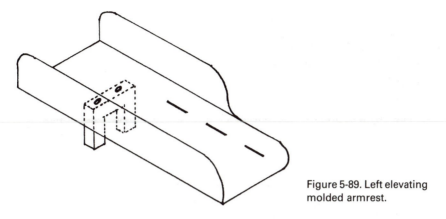

Figure 5-89. Left elevating molded armrest.

elevation of the armrest. The closer the bridge is placed to the hand the lower the elevation.

3. The length of the straps needed to tightly secure the elevating armrest to the wheelchair will need to be increased.

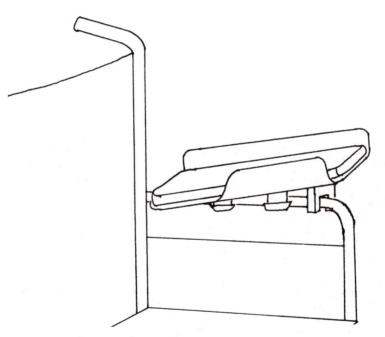

Figure 5-90. Left elevating molded armrest.

Otto Bock Armrests (Otto Bock)

The Otto Bock armrest can be used for most positioning problems of the upper extremity. It is easily adjusted to meet individual needs.

Using the elevating swivel unit, the armrest can be inclined 12 or 25 degrees for control of hand oedema.

Leaving the swivel unit unlocked permits the armrests to swing freely, thus accommodating the upper extremity and the client's body movements. This is an advantage for the spastic extremity as it tends to remain on the armrest and for the client with perceptual deficits as the affected extremity will stay within the immediate visual field.

Otto Bock offers a wide selection of armrests:

—The channel armrest is a one piece unit which provides support to the forearm, but very little for the hand. It is available in one size only.

—The modular channel armrest features a two-piece arm pad concept which allows three sizes of forearm section to be combined with four different types of hand pad. The forearm pad can be used without the hand pad for custom mounting or to promote the use of the hand. The four types of hand pad are:

   a. Flat hand pad: available in two sizes large and medium. The flat hand pad is used for the weak or flaccid hand which does not have flexion contractures.

   b. Palm extensor modular hand pad: available in one size. Specify right or left. It is designed to provide hand support with the fingers in slight flexion. It should not be used if fingers are held in flexion due to spasticity and/or flexion contractures.

   c. Cone-type modular hand pad: available in one size. Specify right or left. For the upper extremity with mild spasticity, it provides positioning for hand and fingers with the forearm held in the mid-position.

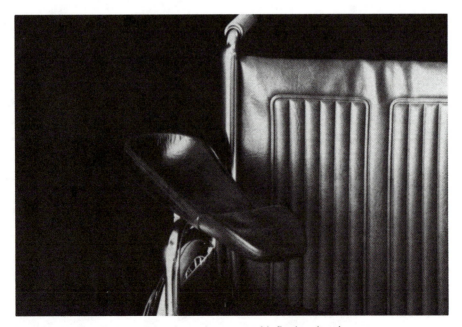

Figure 5-91. Otto Bock modular channel armrest with flat hand pad.

d. Horn type modular hand pad: available in one size. Specify right or left. It provides good support for the spastic upper extremity by allowing additional fingers and hand support with the forearm pronated.

The mounting hardware, the elevating/swivel unit, can be fitted to any type of wheelchair and armrest.

In order to find the appropriate position for the armrest on the wheelchair:

—The client is seated in the wheelchair and the armrest pad is removed.

—The Otto Bock is mounted on the wheelchair armrest frame.

—The swivel unit is unlocked, allowing the armrest to move freely.

—The upper extremity is placed on the armrest.

—The elevating/swivel unit can be moved forward or back to determine the position that provides the most comfortable support for the upper extremity, especially for the shoulder. To confirm the fit, check the client's sitting posture.

—When the most appropriate position is found the elevating/swivel unit is tightly secured to the wheelchair armrest frame. The swivel unit may be locked into one position or left to swing freely.

Wheelchair Table:

The wheelchair table can be used for any positioning problem of the upper extremity. It provides good support and permits the affected upper extremity to stay within the immediate visual field.

It can also assist the client to maintain the upright position.

A clear plastic wheelchair table will not obstruct the lower extremities from the visual field and will help to maintain body awareness.

A wheelchair table facilitates meal management and table activities, but will interfere with the ability to transfer independently.

It may also restrict independent wheelchair mobility with the nonaffected upper extremity.

Wheelchair tables can be fitted to any type of adult wheelchair with full length armrests.

Construction:

Wooden Wheelchair Table

Use 0.5 cm. (1/4 in.) plywood and 1 cm. x 1.5 cm. (0.5 in. x 0.75 in.) wooden strips.

1. To fit a 46 cm. (18 in.) wide adult wheelchair or a 41 cm. (16 in.) wide wheelchair, cut the following pieces:
2. pieces 2 and 3 are glued and nailed to piece 1.
3. Make two straps with 5 cm. (2 in.) wide velcro. The strap is made of one piece 30 cm. (12 in.) long loop and 7.5 cm. (3 in.) long hook. The straps are stapled to the wheelchair table.
4. Wooden wheelchair table should be sanded and varnished for a good finish and for ease of cleaning.

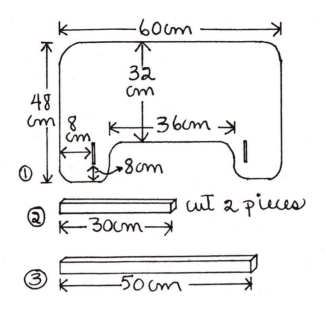

Figure 5-92. On piece 1, make 2 slots of 1 cm. × 5 cm. (0.5 in. × 2 in.)

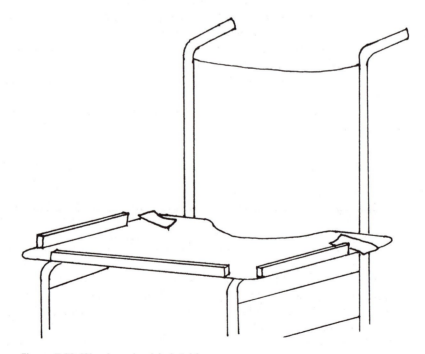

Figure 5-93. Wooden wheelchair table.

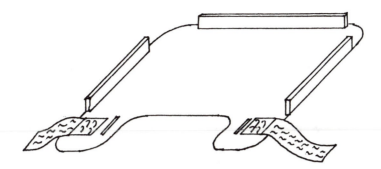

Figure 5-94. Wooden wheelchair table.

Clear Lap Tray (Special Health Systems)

The SHS clear lap tray is available in one standard size to fit any adult wheelchair 41 cm. (16 in.) wide and 46 cm. (18 in.) wide with full length armrests. It is attached to the wheelchair armrests with two velcro straps.

The clear lap tray has a removable rubber trim to encourage awareness of the edge of the tray.

The clear lap tray has the advantage of permitting the client to see the lower extremities thus providing greater body awareness.

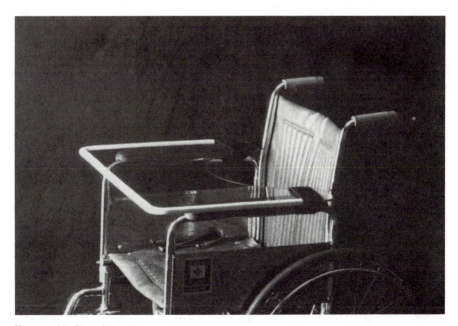

Figure 5-95. Clear lap tray.

Follow Up

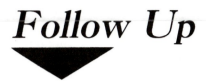

Clients take time to adjust to a new sitting position. The length of time will vary according to the situation.

A new technique or device should be tried in the morning and early in the week to allow for good follow-up. If the client is positioned on a Friday and left for the weekend without monitoring, potential problems could arise.

When many caregivers are involved with a client, labelling a device clearly to indicate the way it should be positioned on the wheelchair is vital to its successful use.

Once a satisfactory position is determined, check the client:

1. the first day—at noon and in the late afternoon
2. the first week—twice a day—once in the morning—to make sure the device is applied correctly, and again after a few hours to observe the effects of fatigue
3. once a week for the first month
4. every six months, or whenever there is a major change in the client's physical status.

Good follow-up is an integral part of the positioning process and will ensure success.

Conclusion

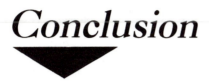

Adaptive seating should be considered an extension of the individual treatment program, and as such should support the goals of the treatment plan. Careful assessment of the needs of the client, combined with the knowledge of available adaptive equipment, will lead to good positioning. Local dealers who specialize in medical equipment are often helpful in locating appropriate devices.

Since each client is unique, there are no predetermined solutions for specific diagnosis or categories. Positioning, therefore, requires time and patience. Several ideas may be tried before the most appropriate solution is found.

The importance of seating intervention in care facilities has to be recognized because almost all aspects of the client's waking life are affected by positioning in a wheelchair.

"Now am I seated as my soul delights..."

Shakespeare; Henry VI

References

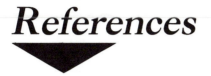

1. Beck, M.A., Klayman, Callahan D., "Impact of Institutionalization on the Posture of Chronic Schizophrenic Patients," American Journal of Occupational Therapy, 34 (5), 332–335, May 1980.
2. Bradey, E., et al., "A Validity Study of Guidelines for Wheelchair Selection," Canadian Journal of Occupational Therapy, 53 (1), 19–24, February 1986.
3. Braile, L.E., "Support for the Drooping Head," American Journal of Occupational Therapy, 35 (10), 661–662, October 1981.
4. Crewe, R.A., "Wheelchair Choice," British Journal of Occupational Therapy, 272–274, November 1979.
5. Everest and Jennings, Inc., "Measuring the Patient," Wheelchair Prescriptions, copyright, April 1979.
6. Fourth International Seating Symposium Syllabus, "Challenges '88: Seating the Disabled," Sunny Hill Hospital, University of British Columbia, University of Tennessee, 1988.
7. G.F. Strong Rehabilitation Center, "Wheelchair Handbook," Canada, 1980.
8. Gilewich, G.,, Paterson, J.S., "Hemiplegic Armrest," Canadian Journal of Occupational Therapy, 42 (2), 63–65, Summer 1975.
9. Gillot, H., et al., "Current Thinking on Pressure Sores," British Journal of Occupational Therapy, 46 (2), 41–43, February 1983.
10. Johnson, Taylor S., "Evaluating the Client With Physical Disabilities for Wheelchair Seating," American Journal of Occupational Therapy, 41 (11), 711–716, November 1987.
11. Kamenetz, H., "The Wheelchair Book: Mobility for the Disabled," Springfield, Illinois, Charles C Thomas, 1969.
12. Lewis, J., "How to Select the Right Wheelchair For You," Accent on Living, 64–70, Summer 1975.
13. Lewis, J., "Five Tips for Successful Wheelchair Fitting," Patient Aid Digest, 18–20, November–December 1975.
14. Lipton, Garber S., Krouskop, T.A., Carter, R.E., "A System for Clinically Evaluating Wheelchair Pressure-Relief Cushions," American Journal of Occupational Therapy, 32 (9), 565–570, October 1978.
15. Lipton, Garber S., "A Classification of Wheelchair Seating," American Journal of Occupational Therapy, 33 (10), 652–654, October 1979.
16. Lipton, Garber S., "Wheelchair Cushions: A Historical Review," American Journal of Occupational Therapy, 39 (7), 453–459, July 1985.

17. O'Brien, M., Tsurumi, K., "The Effect of Two Body Positions on Head Righting in Severely Disabled Individuals With Cerebral Palsy," American Journal of Occupational Therapy, 37 (10), 673–680, October 1983.

18. Otto Bock Orthopedic Industry of Canada, Ltd., "Please, Be Seated! Current Trends for the Disabled," second edition, first printing, Canada 1987.

19. Steed, A., "Using the Steed Cushion in the Treatment of Flaccid Hemiplegia," British Journal of Occupational Therapy, 49 (2), 34–38, February 1986.

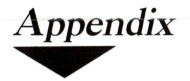

Appendix

List of Manufacturers and Distributors

The following is a list of the manufacturers and distributors for the wheelchairs, seating systems, and adaptations described in this manual.

When ordering a seating system or a wheelchair adaptation, it should be verified that the device is compatible with the wheelchair being used. If an adaptation is required for a special type or size of wheelchair, it is often possible to have items custom-made by the manufacturer.

Everest and Jennings Canadian, Ltd.
111 Snidercroft Road
Toronto, Ontario
L4K 1B6
Canada

Everest and Jennings, Inc.
1803 Pontius Avenue
Los Angeles, California 90025
United States

IDC Tectonics, Ltd.
P.O. Box 2104
Station B
St. Catherines, Ontario
L2M 6P5
Canada

Jay Medical, Ltd.
805 Walnut
Boulder, Colorado 80302
United States

J.T. Posey Co., Inc.
5635 Peck Road
Arcadia, California 91006
United States

Maddack, Inc.
Pequannock, New Jersey 07440
United States

Otto Bock Orthopedic Industry of Canada, Ltd.
251 Saulteaux Crescent
Winnipeg, Manitoba
R3J 3C7
Canada

Otto Bock Orthopedic Industry
4130 Highway 55
Minneapolis, Minnesota 55422
United States

QA2 Seating System
Distributor: Anamed Medical Supply
            Medical Gas
            118 South East Marine Drive
            Vancouver, British Columbia
            V5X 2S3
            Canada

Roho, Inc.
P.O. Box 658
Belleville, Illinois 62222
United States

Special Health Systems
for technical information, you can write to:
  Special Health Systems, Ltd.
  225 Industrial Parkway South
  Aurora, Ontario L4G 3V5
  Canada

Special Health Systems is distributed by:
  Everest and Jennings Canadian, Ltd.
  111 Snidercroft Road
  Toronto, Ontario
  L4K 1B6
  Canada